WEEKEND
WEIGHT-LOSS
DIET

The Juice Lady's

WEEKEND WEIGHT-LOSS DIET

Cherie Calbom, MS, CN

SILOAM

Most CHARISMA HOUSE BOOK GROUP products are available at special quantity discounts for bulk purchase for sales promotions, premiums, fund-raising, and educational needs. For details, write Charisma House Book Group, 600 Rinehart Road, Lake Mary, Florida 32746, or telephone (407) 333-0600.

THE JUICE LADY'S WEEKEND WEIGHT-LOSS DIET by Cherie Calbom
Published by Siloam
Charisma Media/Charisma House Book Group
600 Rinehart Road
Lake Mary, Florida 32746
www.charismahouse.com

Visit the author's website at www.cheriecalbom.com.

Library of Congress Cataloging-in-Publication Data:

Calbom, Cherie.

The juice lady's weekend weight-loss diet / Cherie Calbom.

   p. cm.

Includes bibliographical references (p.   ).

ISBN 978-1-61638-656-6 (trade paper) -- ISBN 978-1-61638-704-4 (e-book) 1. Reducing diets. 2. Vegetable juices. 3. Fruit juices. 4. Detoxification (Health). I. Title.
RM222.2.C228 2012

613.2'5--dc23

                        2011040967

This book contains the opinions and ideas of its author. It is solely for informational and educational purposes and should not be regarded as a substitute for professional medical treatment. The nature of your body's health condition is complex and unique. Therefore, you should consult a health professional before you begin any new exercise, nutrition, or supplementation program or if you have questions about your health. Neither the author nor the publisher shall be liable or responsible for any loss or damage allegedly arising from any information or suggestion in this book.

The statements in this book about consumable products or food have not been evaluated by the Food and Drug Administration. The recipes in this book are to be followed exactly as written. The publisher is not responsible for your specific health or allergy needs that may require medical supervision. The publisher is not responsible for any adverse reactions to the consumption of food or products that have been suggested in this book.

While the author has made every effort to provide accurate telephone numbers and Internet addresses at the time of publication, neither the publisher nor the author assumes any responsibility for errors or for changes that occur after publication.

12 13 14 15 16 — 9 8 7 6 5 4 3 2
Printed in the United States of America

Contents

The Jump-Start Juice Diet That Works!

FRUSTRATED BY DIETS that require months of calorie counting, weighing, and measuring with all sorts of equipment, special foods, expensive pills, or complicated recipes with hard-to-find ingredients? *The Juice Lady's Weekend Weight-Loss Diet* is a simple two-day approach to weight loss. Use it to lose a dress size, get rid of that muffin top, shed a few unwanted pounds, detoxify your body, or jump-start your long-term weight-loss goals. In just two days, you can accomplish any of these objectives by following the plan outlined in this book.

But here's a little secret. The Weekend Weight-Loss Diet really isn't a diet. *It's a fast track to a whole new way of life!* It's the way of eating that I've followed for more than two decades. I know it works. It's how I've maintained my weight. It's worked for hundreds of people whom I've worked with as a nutritionist and the Juice Lady. I became the Juice Lady in 1991 when I went to work for the Juiceman Company while I was finishing my master of science degree at Bastyr University. Since graduating in 1991, I've spoken to audiences, both large and small, at halls, restaurants, meeting rooms, convention centers, churches, and universities. I've taught cooking, juicing, nutrition, and weight-loss classes for many years. Thousands of people have lost weight and improved their health by applying what they've learned in my seminars, classes, and groups.

The juicing program has been proven to facilitate weight loss in university studies, which you'll read more about later on. Now you can enjoy the weight-loss benefits of juicing along with abundant energy, better mood, and improved health.

With a two-day menu plan and scores of scrumptious recipes, you're on your way to a new you! You can enjoy many delicious vegetable juices while melting away fat. That's all you have to do. Just think; you can drink delicious vegetable juices and lose weight!

The Juice Lady's Weekend Weight-Loss Diet is fun, easy, and healthy. It gets fast results without struggle or deprivation—without cravings or climbing the kitchen wall. You will feel satisfied after drinking the fresh vegetable juices. And you will be smiling when you step on the bathroom scale.

But beyond shedding a few pounds quickly, my hope is that this weekend program will put you on the fast track to a whole new lifestyle. The Weekend Weight-Loss Diet is mentioned in my books *The Juice Lady's Turbo Juice Diet* and *The Juice Lady's Living Foods Revolution*. Those books contain longer eating programs that you can incorporate into your daily life for long-lasting results. But the Weekend Weight-Loss program is a simple program I've been recommending for years as a way to jump-start your healthy eating goals. It takes only two days, but it works so well because it feeds the body an abundance of vitamins, minerals, enzymes, and phytonutrients in the form of freshly made juices and high-water content, alkaline plant foods such as vegetables, low-sugar fruit, and sprouts.

And listen up! This is a proven program. It is based on scientific studies that you will learn more about as you read on, which confirm that drinking two glasses of veggie juice daily increased weight loss four times over those who drank no juice.

With this diet you will have a chance to truly feed your body. When you are satisfied nutritionally, your cravings fade away like mist before the sun. Your body can use everything you eat. Very little gets stored up in fat cells. A lot of those little "storage tanks" won't be needed much longer.

Chock-full of nutrients, the vegetable juice combinations in the Weekend Weight-Loss Diet send a signal to the brain that your body is well fed. You will be less likely to experience hunger signals that cause you to clean out the fridge after dinner because your body is still starving for nutrients. And because the juices are rich in antioxidants that bind to toxins and carry them off, they help detoxify the stuff that is a major source of weight gain—toxins and acids. Not only have many people lost weight on the same juice recipes I've included in the Weekend Weight-Loss Diet, but they've also soon discovered they want to keep on feeding their bodies this way because they feel so great—like having abundant energy, better sleep, and a happier state of mind. There are many testimonies and stories on my website www.juiceladyinfo.com.

One story I want to share with you before we go any further is my own. My life drastically changed years ago when I discovered the healing power of freshly made juice and raw and whole foods. I'd like to share my story with you.

I WONDERED IF I WOULD EVER BE WELL AGAIN

When I turned thirty, I had to quit my job. I had chronic fatigue syndrome and fibromyalgia that made me so sick I couldn't work. I felt as though I had a never-ending flu. Constantly feverish with swollen glands and perennially lethargic, I was also in constant pain. My body ached as though I'd been bounced around in a washing machine.

I had moved back to my father's home in Colorado to try and recover. But not one doctor had an answer as to what I should do to facilitate healing. I read about juicing and whole foods, and it made sense. So I bought a juicer and designed a program I could follow.

I juiced and ate a nearly perfect diet of live and whole foods for three months. There were ups and downs throughout. I had days where I felt encouraged that I was making some progress but other days where I felt worse. Those were discouraging and made me wonder if health was the elusive dream. No one told me about detox reactions, which was what I was experiencing. I was obviously very toxic, and my body was cleansing away all that stuff that had made me sick. This caused some not-so-good days amid the promising ones.

But one morning I woke up early—early for me, which was around 8:00 a.m.—without an alarm sounding off. I felt like someone had given me a new body in the night. I had so much energy I actually wanted to go jogging. What had happened? This new sensation of health had just appeared with the morning sun. But actually my body had been healing all along; it just had not manifested until that day. What a wonderful sense of being alive! I looked and felt completely renewed.

With my juicer in tow and a new lifestyle fully embraced, I returned to Southern California a couple weeks later to finish writing my first book. For nearly a year it was "ten steps forward" with great health and more energy and stamina than I'd ever remembered.

Then, all of a sudden, I took a giant step back.

THE EVENT THAT TOOK MY BREATH AWAY

July fourth was a beautiful day like so many others in Southern California. I celebrated the holiday with friends that evening at a backyard barbecue. I returned just before midnight to the house I was sitting for vacationing friends and crawled into bed.

I woke up shivering some time later. "Why is it so cold?" I wondered as I rolled over to see the clock; it was 3:00 a.m. That's when I noticed that the door to the backyard was open. Then I noticed him crouched in the shadows of the corner of the room—a shirtless young guy in shorts. I blinked twice, trying to deny what I was seeing.

Instead of running, he leaped off the floor and ran toward me. He pulled a pipe from his shorts and began attacking me, beating me repeatedly over the head and yelling, "Now you are dead!" We fought, or I should say I tried to defend myself and grab the pipe. It finally flew out of his hands. That's when he choked me to unconsciousness. I felt life leaving my body. In those last few seconds, I knew I was dying. "This is it, the end of my life," I thought. I felt sad for the people who loved me and how they would feel about this tragic event. Then I felt my spirit leave in a sensation of popping out of my body and floating upward. Suddenly everything was peaceful and still. I sensed I was traveling, at what seemed like the speed of light, through black space. I saw what seemed like lights twinkling in the distance.

But all of a sudden I was back in my body, outside the house, clinging to a fence at the end of the dog run. I don't know how I got there. I screamed for help with all the breath I had. Each time I screamed, I passed out and landed on the cement. I then had to pull myself up again. But finally a neighbor heard me and sent her husband to help. Within a short time I was on my way to the hospital.

Lying on a cold gurney at 4:30 a.m., chilled to the bone, in and out of consciousness, I tried to assess my injuries, which was virtually impossible. The next thing I knew, I was being wheeled off to surgery. Later I learned that I had suffered serious injuries to my head, neck, back, and right hand, with multiple head wounds and part of my scalp torn from my head. I also incurred numerous cracked teeth that resulted in several root canals and crowns months later.

My right hand sustained the most severe injuries, with two knuckles crushed to mere bone fragments that had to be held together by three metal pins. Six months after the attack I still couldn't use it. The cast I wore—with bands holding up the ring finger, which had almost been torn from my hand, and various odd-shaped molded parts—looked like something from a science-fiction movie. I felt and looked worse than hopeless, with a shaved top of my head, totally red and swollen eyes, a gash on my face, a useless right hand, terrorizing fear, and barely enough energy to get dressed in the morning.

I was an emotional wreck. I couldn't sleep at night—not even a minute. It was torturous. I'd lie in bed all night and stare at the ceiling or the bedroom door. I had five lights that I kept on all night. I'd try to read, but my eyes would sting. I could sleep for only a little while during the day.

But the worst part was the pain in my soul that nearly took my breath away. All the emotional pain of the attack joined up with the pain and trauma of my past for an emotional tsunami. My past had been riddled with loss, trauma, and anxiety. My brother died when I was two. My mother had died of cancer when I was six. I couldn't remember much about her death—the memories seemed blocked. But my cousin said I fainted at her funeral. That told me the impact was huge.

As you can probably imagine, wrapped in my soul was a significant amount of anguish and pain. It took every ounce of my will, faith, and trust in God, deep spiritual work, alternative medical help, extra vitamins and minerals, vegetable juicing, emotional release, healing prayer, and numerous detox programs to heal physically, mentally, and emotionally. I met a nutritionally minded physician who had healed his own slow-mending broken bones with lots of vitamin-mineral IVs. He gave me similar IVs. Juicing, cleansing, nutritional supplements, a nearly perfect diet, prayer, and physical therapy helped my bones and other injuries heal.

After following this regimen for about nine months, what my hand surgeon said would be impossible became real—a fully restored, fully functional hand. He had told me I'd never use my right hand again and that it wasn't even possible to put in plastic knuckles because of its poor condition. But my knuckles did indeed re-form primarily through prayer, and function of my hand returned. A day came when he told me I was completely healed, and though he admitted he didn't believe in miracles, he said, "You're the closest thing I've seen to one."

It was a miracle! I had a useful hand again, and my career in writing was not over as I thought it would be. My inner wounds were what seemed severest in the end and the hardest to heal. Nevertheless, they mended too. I experienced healing from the painful memories and trauma of the attack and the wounds from the past through prayer, laying on of hands, and deep emotional healing work.

I called them the *kitchen angels*—the ladies who prayed for me around their kitchen table week after week until my soul was healed. I cried endless buckets of tears that had been pent up in my soul. It all needed release. Forgiveness and letting go came in stages and was an integral part of my total healing. I had to be honest about what I really felt and willing to face the pain and toxic emotions confined inside, and then let them go. Finally, one day after a long journey—I felt free. A time came when I could celebrate the Fourth of July without fear.

When I look back to that first day in the hospital after many hours of surgery, it's amazing to me that I made it. My hand was resting in a sling hanging above my head. It was wrapped with so much stuff it looked like George Foreman's boxing glove. My face was black and blue and my eyes were red—no whites—they were completely red. As I lay there alone with tears streaming down my face, I asked God if He could bring something good out of this horrific situation. I needed something to hang onto. My prayer was answered. Eventually I knew my purpose was to love people to life through my writing and nutritional information to help them find their way to health and healing. If I could recover from all that had happened to me, they could too. No matter what anyone faced, there was hope.

I have a juice recipe called "You Are Loved Cocktail" in this book. I named it that because I want you to know that you are loved, that I send you my love between the lines of this book and with the juice and raw food recipes. There is hope for you, no matter what health challenges you face. There's a purpose for your life, just as there was for mine. You need to be strong and well to complete your purpose. You can be greatly served by a positive mind and an optimistic attitude. To that end *The Juice Lady's Weekend Weight-Loss Diet* can help you live your life to the fullest and to finish well.

A New Way of Life

When you complete the Weekend Weight-Loss Diet, my hope is that you will have started a change in your eating habits. The cravings and urges that once lured you to snack foods you didn't even want are starting to disappear. Yo-yo dieting could be gone forever—if you make this style of eating your way of life.

Best of all—you will be healthier. Just as in the success stories people share with me daily through letters and e-mails, you too may experience more weight-loss success, coupled with energy and abundant health, than you have ever thought possible. You can have a happier mood and the opportunity to enjoy each day. And you will stand the greatest chance of preventing serious diseases such as cancer, diabetes, or heart disease.

This diet is your first step to a new way of life you will want to stick with because feeling healthy, happy, and energetic is something you will never want to lose once you attain it—no matter how alluring some foods might be. So lift your glass of veggie juice and toast to a new era in your life!

Chapter 1

Weight Loss on a Mission

THE WORLD HEALTH Organization estimates that by 2015, there will be more than 1.5 billion overweight consumers, incurring health costs beyond $117 billion per year in the US alone.[1] It's obvious that we need to do something differently. We need a new way of life—a revolution in how we eat, one that we adopt for the rest of our lives.

What if you found a weight-loss program that could help you lose weight more effectively than anything you've ever tried? And what if that program didn't involve expensive meals you had to order, pills you had to buy, or anything other than great whole foods you prepare in your kitchen? What if that program helped you look and feel better than ever? And what if it was such an energizing way of life that you wanted to follow it for the rest of your life? Are you interested?

The Juice Lady's Weekend Weight-Loss Diet is a fast track to just such a program. This two-day jump start can lead you into a transformative lifestyle that is helping thousands of people lose weight, keep it off for good, and completely revolutionize their health. This is what I call *weight loss on a mission*—the mission is to help you become healthy, happy, and filled with life, as well as slim and fit. (You'll find a complete weight-loss juicing program in my book *The Juice Lady's Turbo Diet*.)

Freshly made vegetable juices are at the center of the weekend weight-loss diet. They provide concentrated sources of very absorbable nutrients. They are low in fat and calories, so replacing higher-calorie foods with fresh juice is a shoo-in for weight-loss success.

But the benefits of juicing don't stop there. Vegetable juices help curb cravings because they satisfy your body's nutrient needs. They're alkaline, which is very helpful to balance out a system that's most probably too acidic. They're also high in antioxidants that are antiaging and immune enhancing—that means you're giving your body the things it needs to start looking and feeling younger.

Fresh Juice—a Cornucopia of Nutrients

Every time you pour a glass of juice, picture a cornucopia of nutrients cascading into your body, promoting health, revving up your metabolism, balancing weight, and increasing vitality. This mélange of nutrients can change your life—completely change your life—as it completely changed mine! Here's what every glass of juice provides.

Amino acids

Did you ever consider juice to be a source of protein? Most people would say no. Surprisingly, it does offer more amino acids than you might think. We use amino acids to form muscles, ligaments, tendons, hair, nails, and skin. Protein is needed to create enzymes, which direct chemical reactions, and hormones, which guide bodily functions. Fruits and vegetables contain lower quantities of protein than animal foods such as muscle meats and dairy products. Therefore they are thought of as poor protein sources. But juices are concentrated forms of vegetables and so provide easily absorbed amino acids, the building blocks that make up protein. For example, 16 ounces of carrot juice (2–3 pounds of carrots) provides about 5 grams of protein (the equivalent of about a chicken wing or 2 ounces of tofu). I don't recommend drinking that much carrot juice because of the sugar content, but that's an example.

Vegetable protein is not complete protein, so it does not provide all the amino acids your body needs. In addition to lots of dark leafy greens, when you finish your weekend weight-loss kick start, you'll want to eat other protein sources, such as sprouts, legumes (beans, lentils, and split peas), nuts, seeds, and whole grains. If you're not vegan, you can add eggs and free-range, grass-fed muscle meats such as chicken, turkey, lamb, and beef along with wild-caught fish.

Carbohydrates

Most vegetable juice contains good carbohydrates. The exceptions would be carrots and beets, which have higher sugar content. They should be used in small quantities and diluted with low-sugar vegetable juices such as cucumber and dark leafy greens. Carbs provide fuel for the body, which it uses for energy, heat production, and chemical reactions. The chemical bonds of carbohydrates lock in the energy a plant takes up from the sun and soil, and this energy is released when the body burns plant food as fuel.

There are three categories of carbs: simple (sugars), complex (starches and fiber), and fiber. Choose more complex carbohydrates in your diet than simple carbs. There are more simple sugars in fruit juice than vegetable juice, which is why I recommend you juice primarily vegetables, use low-sugar fruit for flavor and a little sweetness, and in most cases drink no more than 4 ounces of fruit juice a day.

Both insoluble fiber and soluble fiber are found in whole fruits and vegetables—both types are needed for good health. It's amazing how many people still say juice doesn't have any fiber. It contains the soluble form—pectin and gums, which are excellent for the digestive tract. Soluble fiber also helps to lower cholesterol, stabilize blood sugar, and improve good bowel bacteria and elimination.

Essential fatty acids

There is very little fat in fruit and vegetable juices, but the fats juice does contain are essential to your health. The essential fatty acids (EFAs)—linoleic and alpha-linolenic acids in particular—found in fresh juice function as components of nerve cells, cellular membranes, and hormonelike substances called prostaglandins. They are also required for energy production.

Vitamins

Fresh juice is replete with vitamins, but heat and processing destroy vitamins. We need these organic substances because they take part, along with minerals and enzymes, in chemical reactions throughout the body. For example, vitamin C participates in the production of collagen, one of the main types of protein found in the body that keeps your skin looking fresh and youthful rather than sagging and aging. Fresh juices are excellent sources of water-soluble vitamins such as C, many of the B vitamins, and some fat-soluble vitamins such as E and K, along with key phytonutrients like beta-carotene (known as pro-vitamin A), lutein, lycopene, and zeaxanthin. They also are coupled with cofactors that increase the effectiveness of each nutrient; for example, vitamin C and bioflavonoids work together synergistically to make each more effective.

Minerals

There are about two dozen minerals that your body needs to function well, and they're abundant in fresh juice. They make up part of bones, teeth, and blood, and they help maintain normal cellular function. The major minerals include calcium, chloride, magnesium, phosphorus, potassium, sodium, and sulfur. Trace minerals, which include boron, chromium, cobalt, copper, manganese, nickel, selenium, vanadium, and zinc, are those needed in very small amounts.

Minerals occur in inorganic forms in the soil, and plants

incorporate them into their tissues. As a part of this process, the minerals are combined with organic molecules into easily absorbable forms, which makes plants an excellent dietary source of minerals. Juicing is believed to provide even better mineral absorption than whole vegetables because the process of juicing releases minerals into a highly absorbable, easily digestible form.

Enzymes

These living molecules are prevalent in raw foods, but heat, such as cooking and pasteurization, destroys them. Enzymes facilitate the biochemical reactions necessary for life. They are complex structures composed predominantly of protein and usually require additional cofactors to function, including vitamins; minerals such as calcium, magnesium, and iron; and other elements. Fresh juice is chock-full of enzymes. Without them we would not have life.

When you eat and drink enzyme-rich foods, these little molecules help break down food in the digestive tract, thereby sparing the pancreas, liver, and stomach—the body's enzyme producers—from overwork. This sparing action is known as the "law of adaptive secretion of digestive enzymes," which asserts that the body will adapt or change the amount of digestive enzymes it produces according to what is needed. According to this law, when a portion of the food you eat is digested by enzymes present in the food, the body won't need to secrete as much of its own enzymes. This allows the body's energy to be shifted from digestion to other functions such as repair and rejuvenation.

Fresh juices require very little energy expenditure to digest. That is one reason why people who start consistently drinking fresh veggie juice often report that their digestion and elimination improve and that they feel better and more energized right away.

Phytochemicals

Plants contain substances know as phytochemicals that protect them from disease, injury, and pollution. *Phyto* means plant, and *chemical* in this context means nutrient. There are tens of thousands of phytochemicals in the foods we eat. For example, the average tomato may contain up to ten thousand different types of these nutrients, with one of the most famous being lycopene. Phytochemicals give plants their color, odor, and flavor. Unlike vitamins and enzymes, they are heat stable and can withstand cooking. Some of them, such as lycopene, appear to be more effective when cooked.

Biophotons

There's one more substance abundant in raw foods that is more difficult to measure than the others. It's known as biophotons, which is light energy that is found in the living cells of raw plant foods. These photons have been shown to emit coherent light energy when uniquely photographed (Kirlian photography). This light energy is believed to have many benefits when consumed, such as aiding cellular communication and feeding the mitochondria and the DNA. They are believed to contribute to our energy, vitality, and a feeling of vibrancy and well-being.

Now that you've learned about the powerful nutritional punch packed inside each glass of juice you drink, let's consider how this applies to weight loss.

POWER FOODS THAT GIVE YOUR WEIGHT LOSS A BIG BOOST

In addition to some of the basic steps you can take to achieve weight-loss success, there are specific foods you can add to your weight-loss program that will make a huge difference in assisting your body in burning fat. These super foods can help you succeed and give you super-size health dividends at the same time. Be sure to add them to your weight-loss program.

Green juice: the number one fat cure. In honor of his hundredth show, Dr. Oz served on the set his favorite green juice drink to one hundred people who had lost thirteen thousand pounds combined. This blend of cucumbers, apple, and leafy greens started a new wave of interest in green juices for weight loss. So why do green juices work so well? Dr. Oz cites the fact that they compensate for the fact that most of us are simply not getting sufficient nourishment from standard diets. He says, "We know we have to have at least five fistfuls of leafy green vegetables and fruit every day, so we make a morning green drink."[2]

There's evidence to suggest that even if we took the time to chew up five cups of green veggies each day, we wouldn't get as much benefit from them as we would from juicing them. The mechanical process of juicing the vegetables breaks apart plant cell walls and makes absorption better than even when the best "chewers" chew their food at least thirty times before swallowing. It has an effect like throwing marbles at a chain-link fence rather than tennis balls; their contents are going to go through in a way that tennis balls can't.

The juices contain easily absorbed micronutrients that will do more than slim you down—they'll optimize your overall health and wellness. There's science behind the green juices transformative powers and a number of reasons why the juices, along with a high intake of living foods, energize your body, fire up your metabolism, speed slimming, and overhaul your health. Here's the evidence as to why it works.

Green Veggies Help Lower the Risk of Type 2 Diabetes

Because of their high magnesium content and low glycemic index, green leafy vegetables are also valuable for persons with type 2 diabetes. One study revealed that an increase of just one and one-half servings a day of green leafy vegetables was associated with a 14 percent lower risk of diabetes.[3]

Magnesium-rich greens ramp up your energy. A British study comparing the metabolism of female twins found that magnesium intake was *the most important* dietary variable that determined adiponectin levels.[4] Adiponectin is a fat cell hormone that promotes insulin sensitivity. This hormone has recently gained attention from researchers because of its regulation of glucose and fat metabolism. Elevated levels of adiponectin are associated with increased insulin sensitivity and fat burning. Adiponectin also seems to work closely with leptin—a hormone that helps control the appetite. As you lose weight, this hormone gets a boost. Fresh fruit and vegetables have a positive influence on this hormone, which is made in fat cells. It boosts metabolism and helps regulate inflammation, which, consequently, helps to prevent weight gain, becoming a type 2 diabetic, or developing heart disease.

This new study shows very clearly that adequate magnesium is imperative to maintaining adiponectin levels. This means that a deficiency of magnesium, which is common in America, is a clear contributor to the problems people have with weight management. Magnesium also plays a key role in fighting off stress and anxiety, supporting restful sleep, preventing restless leg syndrome, and boosting energy.

Further, magnesium helps prevent fat storage. When magnesium is low, cells fail to recognize insulin. As a result, glucose accumulates in the blood—and then it gets stored as fat instead of being burned for fuel.

Green plants, which are rich in magnesium, are far superior to magnesium supplements because the supplements' particles are a bit large for the body to entirely absorb. (I'm in favor of taking magnesium supplements, if they are needed, but as an adjunct to a magnesium-rich diet.) Green plants take inorganic minerals from the soil through their tiny roots and incorporate them into their cells. They become organic particles that are much smaller and easier for the body to absorb. It is estimated that more than 90 percent of a plant's minerals is delivered to the cells when you juice the greens. So juice up those leaves—chard, collards, beet tops, parsley, spinach—the five highest in magnesium, plus kohlrabi leaves, kale, dandelion greens, lettuce, and mustard greens.

Here's the good news—you'll increase your energy with this high-octane fuel! That means you'll get more done and feel more like working out, so you'll burn more calories and build more muscle.

Enzymes Speed Fat Burning

Our bodies produce enzymes that are used in digesting the food we eat. They can be found in the saliva, small intestine, stomach, liver, and pancreas. These hardworking little catalysts break down proteins, fats, and carbohydrates into fatty acids, amino acids, and forms of glucose that feed your cells.

Enzymes are responsible for a host of reactions in the body. All the minerals, herbs, vitamins, and hormones we take can't do their jobs without enzymes. When your diet is deficient in enzymes from live foods (uncooked, not processed), your body has to work harder to produce the enzymes it needs. If you're deficient, you may experience weight gain, depression, and many other maladies that plague modern society.

Enzymes are truly weight-loss supermen. But these magic bullets start decreasing as we age—by age thirty-five most people see a decline in their enzyme production. Still, we need them for weight loss and good digestion. It's enzymes that assist in the breakdown and burning of fat.

This is where juices come to the rescue—as I mentioned earlier, they're packed with enzymes. Eating a high percentage of raw food is important because cooking and processing our food destroys enzymes. When you drink fresh, live juices and eat plenty of living foods, the enzymes they contain kick your metabolism into gear by helping to spare your liver and pancreas from working so hard. Then these organs can focus on their metabolic tasks of burning fat and producing energy. And your digestion will improve. This affects your whole life, your whole being.

Three Super-Hero Enzymes

- *Lipase.* Lipase is a fat-splitting enzyme that is abundant in raw foods. It assists your body in digestion, fat distribution, and fat burning. However, few of us eat enough raw foods to get sufficient lipase to burn even a normal amount of fat, not to mention any excess fat. Without lipase, fat accumulates. You can see it on your hips, thighs, buttocks, and stomach. Lipase is richest in raw foods that contain some fat, such as sprouted seeds and nuts, avocado, and fresh coconut meat.

- *Protease.* As your body burns flab, toxins are released into your system. This can cause water retention and bloating. Protease is a digestive enzyme that helps to break down proteins and eliminate toxins. Eliminating toxins is essential when you're burning fat. If your body is storing toxins, it's very difficult to burn fat. But protease comes to the rescue and attacks and eliminates toxins. So, as you can see, it's crucial to have plenty of protease during weight loss. Protease is richest in the leaves of plants. So juice up those green leaves and burn fat. Plus, the greens are also rich in antioxidants that bind up toxins and carry them out of your system so they won't hurt your cells. That means you'll get double action with green juices.

- *Amylase.* Amylase is a digestive enzyme that breaks down complex carbohydrates into simple sugars. It's also present in saliva. So while we chew our food, it goes to work on carbs. That's why it's recommended that you chew each mouthful of food about thirty times. The pancreas also makes amylase. And amylase is plentiful in seeds that contain starch. (You can juice most seeds of fruits and vegetables.) Its therapeutic use is in regulation of histamine, which is produced in response to recognized invaders to the body. Histamine is a responder in allergic reactions such as hay fever and is what causes hives, itchy watery eyes, sneezing, and runny noses. Amylase breaks down the histamine produced by the body in response to allergens like pollen or dust mites. Some health professionals believe it may help the body identify the allergen as not being harmful so it doesn't produce the histamine in the first place. This is one reason that people on a high raw plant diet often experience improvement in their allergies.

For the most effective approach to increasing enzymes, you may also want to take an enzyme supplement. I especially like an enzyme formula that is taken between meals—it cleans up any undigested particles of food floating around the system and greatly improves digestion. A popular side benefit is that your hair gets thicker and your nails grow stronger. (For more information on these enzymes, see Appendix A.)

Greens Alkalize Your Body and Promote Weight Loss

Many people eat a high-sugar breakfast consisting of foods and drinks such as orange juice, toast, jam, honey, sweetened cereal, sweet rolls, doughnuts, muffins, waffles, or pancakes. All this sugar and simple carbohydrates (which turn to sugar easily) promote acidity and cause yeast and fungus to grow. They also produce a lot of acid. Traditional high-protein breakfast foods such as omelets, cheese, bacon, sausage, and meat promote elevated acid levels in the body as well. Add to that highly acidic drinks such as coffee, black tea, sodas, alcohol, and sports drinks, and acidic foods for lunch and dinner, and you're consuming loads of acid-forming foods throughout the day. Keep in mind that acid-forming food does not mean the state of the food when you eat or drink it but the final ash residue after it is metabolized. As a result of this style of eating, along with not eating enough green veggies and other living foods, many people suffer from a condition known as mild acidosis, which is an out-of-balance pH leaning toward acidity. This means that the body is continually fighting to maintain pH balance.

One of the symptoms of acidosis is weight gain and an inability to lose weight. That's because the body tends to store acid in fat cells and to hang on to those cells to protect your delicate tissues and organs. It will even make more fat cells in which to store acid, if they're needed. To turn this scenario around, it's important to alkalize your body. Greens are one of the best choices you could make because they're very alkaline. And juicing them gives you an easy way to consume a lot more than you could chew up in a day.

To give your body a great start in rebalancing your pH, make 60 percent to 80 percent of your diet alkalizing foods such as green vegetables, raw juices, grasses such as wheatgrass juice, fresh vegetables and fruit, raw seeds, nuts, and sprouts. Greatly limit or avoid your consumption of acid-forming foods such as meat, dairy products, chocolate, sweets, bread and all other yeast products, alcohol, carbonated drinks, sports drinks, coffee, and black tea.

When pH balance is achieved, the body should automatically drop to its ideal, healthy weight unless you have other health challenges. (But those should heal too over time.) As the acidic environment is neutralized with mineral-rich alkaline foods, there will be no need for your body to create new fat cells for storage of acid. And since the remaining fat is no longer needed to store acid wastes, it simply melts away.

This is also a great way to restore your health. Many diseases such as cancer thrive in an acidic state. Take away the acid, and they don't do as well. An alkaline diet also boosts your energy level, improves skin, reduces allergies, sustains the immune system, and enhances mental clarity.

THERMOGENIC FOODS REV UP YOUR METABOLISM

Thermogenesis means the production of heat, which raises metabolism and burns calories. Thermogenic foods are essentially fat-burning foods and spices that help increase your metabolism. This means that with some of your kitchen staples, you can burn off fat during or right after you eat and increase your fat-burning potential just by eating them. So include these super foods often in your juices and recipes.

Hot peppers. Imagine eating hot peppers and revving up your metabolism enough to lose weight. A study in 2010 found that obesity was caused by a lack of thermogenic response in the body rather than by overeating or lack of exercise. "The animals developed obesity mainly because they didn't produce enough heat after eating, not because the animals ate more or were less active," said Dr. Yong Xu, instructor of internal medicine at UT Southwestern and co-lead author of the study.[5] Another study found that hot peppers turn up the internal heat, which helps in burning calories.[6] You can add hot peppers or a dash of hot sauce to many juice recipes or almost any dish and make it taste delicious.

Garlic. When it comes to weight loss, garlic appears to be a miracle food. A team of doctors at Israel's Tel Hashomer Hospital conducted a test on rats to find out how garlic can prevent diabetes and heart attacks, and they found an interesting side effect—none of the rats given allicin (a compound in garlic) gained weight.[7] Garlic is a known appetite suppressant. The strong odor of garlic stimulates the satiety center in the brain, thereby reducing feelings of hunger. It also increases the brain's sensitivity to leptin, a hormone produced by fat cells that controls appetite. Further, garlic stimulates the nervous system to release hormones such as adrenalin, which speed up metabolic rate. This means a greater ability to burn calories. More calories burned means less weight gained—a terrific correlation.

Ginger. Ginger contains a substance that stimulates gastric enzymes, which can boost metabolism. The better your metabolism, the more calories you'll burn. It has been shown to be an anti-inflammatory—inflammation is implicated in obesity. Ginger helps improve gastric motility—the spontaneous peristaltic movements of the stomach that aid in moving food through the digestive system. When the digestive system is functioning at its best, you'll experience less bloating and constipation. It has also been found to lower cholesterol. And ginger is the top vegan source of zinc, which gives a big boost to your immune system. Top that off with the fact that it tastes delicious in juice recipes, and you have a super spice. I add it to almost every juice recipe I make.

Parsley. This dark green herb offers a great way to make your dishes and juices super healthy. Parsley helps you detox because it's chock-full of antioxidants, like vitamin C and flavonoids, and it's loaded with minerals and chlorophyll. It's also a natural diuretic, which helps you get rid of stored water. That means thinner ankles, feet, and fingers. And it improves digestion and strengthens the spleen as well. You can add a handful of parsley to almost any juice recipe and you won't even know it's there.

Cranberries. Studies show that cranberries are loaded with acids that researchers believe are useful in dissolving fat deposits. When fat deposits settle in the body, they are hard to get rid of, so it's best to get them before they get "hooked on" you. Some studies point out that the enzymes in cranberries can aid metabolism, which gives a boost to weight loss.[8] This tart little fruit is a natural diuretic, helping you get rid of excess water and bloating. Of all the fruits, cranberries rank number two for antioxidant content, which helps detoxify the body. And they promote healthy teeth and gums, fight urinary track infections, improve heart health, and keep cancer at bay.

Kathy, who was featured in my "Holiday Fat Buster" article in the December 27, 2010, issue of *Woman's World*, issue, lost 5 pounds in seventy-two hours drinking a cranberry, pear, cucumber, and ginger cocktail along with the rest of the Turbo Juice Diet Program. Within a week Kathy's tummy was down 5.5 inches—she said she had to keep measuring to make sure it was right. Regarding the juice diet program, she said, "Overall, I had a lot of energy and no hunger."[9]

You can add cranberries to many recipes for a delicious enhancer to your juice drinks and a boost to your weight loss at the same time. If you buy these berries when they're in season, you can freeze a few packages to have on hand for seasons when they aren't available.

Blueberries. A 2010 study found that blueberries can help you get rid of belly fat, thanks to the high level of phytochemicals (antioxidants) they contain. The study also showed that blueberries are helpful in preventing type 2 diabetes, and the benefits were even greater when the blueberries were combined with a low-fat diet.[10] Moreover, blueberries can also help fight hardening of the arteries and improve the memory.

Lemons. Adding just a tablespoon of fresh lemon juice to your water, salad, or soup will help ward off cravings, alkalize your body, and keep your insulin levels in check. Hot lemon water with a dash of cayenne pepper is a great way to start your day—it gets the liver, your fat-burning organ, moving in the morning. It's also a natural diuretic and helps clear out toxins from your system. Further, it aids the digestive process and prevents constipation. It can also help alleviate heartburn—just add a tablespoon of fresh lemon juice to water and drink with your meal. Limonene, a compound in lemons, helps short-circuit the production of acid in the stomach—lemons are very alkalizing. Meyer lemons, my favorite, are sweeter and are available in the winter.

THE LOW-GLYCEMIC BENEFITS OF JUICING

The glycemic index has become a popular weight-loss tool based in part on the fact that high-glycemic foods raise blood sugar levels, cause the body to secrete excess insulin, and lead to the storage of fat. Originally developed to help diabetics manage blood sugar control, the glycemic index has become popular in the weight-loss market largely because it works so well. Researchers reported in the *Journal of the American Medical Association* that patients who lost weight with a low-glycemic diet kept the weight off longer than patients who lost the same amount of weight with a low-fat diet.[11]

The glycemic index (GI) diet refers to a system of ranking carbohydrates according to how much a certain amount of each food raises a person's blood sugar level. It's determined by measuring how much a 50-gram serving of carbohydrate raises a person's blood sugar level compared with a control.

Virtually all carbohydrates are digested into glucose and cause a temporary rise in blood glucose levels, called the glycemic response. But some foods raise it more than others. This response is affected by many factors, including the quantity of food, the amount and type of carbohydrate, how it's cooked or eaten raw, and the degree of processing. Each food is assigned an index number from 1 to 100, with 100 as the reference score for pure glucose. Typically, foods are rated high (greater than 70), moderate (56–69), and low (less than 55).

Low-glycemic foods, especially raw carbohydrates, can help control blood sugar, appetite, and weight. Though helpful for everyone, they are especially helpful for people with type 2 diabetes, prediabetes, hypoglycemia, insulin resistance, and metabolic syndrome. Low-glycemic foods are absorbed more slowly, allowing a person to feel full longer and therefore be less likely to overeat. Raw food experts such as Dr. John Douglass have found that raw carbohydrates such as the raw juices are better tolerated than cooked carbs. They don't elicit the addictive cravings that cooked foods cause. Douglass believes, as does the Finish expert A. I. Virtanen, that the enzymes in raw food play an important role in the way they stimulate weight loss as they do in the treatment of obesity.[12]

When you get to chapter 6, "Beyond the Weekend," you will be encouraged to choose most of your carbohydrate foods from the low-glycemic index and a large percentage of those foods as raw. The foods I recommend eating after you've completed your weekend weight-loss diet (see Appendix B) are for the most part low glycemic and are nutrient-rich, not refined, and higher in fiber—like whole vegetables, fruit, and legumes (beans, lentils, split peas).

NOT ALL CARBS ARE CREATED EQUAL

Different carbohydrates take different pathways in the body after digestion. For example, some starchy foods are bound by an outer layer of very complex starches (fiber) like the legumes (beans, lentils, split peas), which increases the time it takes for them to be digested. So even though legumes are relatively high in carbohydrates, they have a lower glycemic response because of their complex encasing.

There is also the antioxidant potential of foods to consider, meaning the amount of antioxidant nutrients a food contains, such as beta-carotene and vitamin C that are abundant in many fruits and vegetables. In Chinese culture, carrots are often used as cooling medicine. Carrots, beets (both very rich in beta-carotene), and other brightly colored vegetables are especially important to include in our diet to prevent disease. These days many health professionals suggest we eliminate carrots and beets because of their glycemic rating, but the weekend weight-loss diet does not exclude them because of their high nutrient and fiber content. But I do recommend that you use them in small amounts because they are higher in sugar.

Also, please keep in mind that not all low-glycemic foods are healthy fare. Low-glycemic foods include candy bars and potato chips. These foods are very nutrient depleted, contain sugar or turn to sugar easily, and lack fiber. You need to get the best nutrition for your choices.

With this plan, there's no obsessing over the glycemic index either, just a basic understanding of the principles. Keep in mind that certain factors can change a score, such as the riper the fruit, the higher the glycemic index score. But always choose ripe fruits and vegetables over unripe; they are healthier by far. Adding good fat to foods can lower the GI score. And keep in mind that the GI response to any given food also varies widely from person to person. It can even vary within the same person from day to day. So it's important to listen to your body and determine how the foods you are eating are affecting you.

More Than Weight Loss

Years ago when I was taking prerequisites for my master of science program in whole foods nutrition at Bastyr University, I worked for a weight-loss center part time as a nutrition counselor. I noticed that a number of people who entered the program looked healthy, meaning they had good skin color and tone and vibrancy—they were just overweight. Soon into the program, I noticed that though they were losing weight, they weren't looking healthier. I observed a loss of skin tone, skin color turning a grayish pallor, and a loss of energy and vitality. I was alarmed. Even as a student I knew that it was not just about dropping weight; it was about getting healthier. I quit the job, unable to promote something that I felt did harm.

When you embark on a weight-loss program, it should be about getting healthier along with losing weight. Whether you want to lose 10, 20, 50, 100, or even 200 pounds, it isn't just about getting the weight off any way you can. I know people who have lost weight through drastic means and ruined their health in the process.

Losing weight with vegetable juices and kicking off your program with the Weekend Weight-Loss Diet is the first step in choosing a weight-loss regimen that doesn't sacrifice your health. That's why I'm excited about introducing you to the Weekend Weight-Loss Diet. I know what it can do for you. So many people have praised this program and my other juice diets because of the increased health and energy they experienced. And if they can experience these great results, you can too. You're off to a great start and a lifetime of fitness!

Chapter 2

Top Ten Roadblocks to Weight Loss

I F YOU'VE TRIED to lose weight and just can't seem to get the scale to budge in spite of your best efforts, or you've reached a weight-loss plateau, you may need a specific intervention that gets to the root of why you aren't losing the weight you want. The good news is that when you correct the issue, you will get healthier, and weight loss may end up being a secondary benefit compared to all the other payoffs.

There are numerous reasons why people can't lose weight that go beyond simply eating too many calories and not exercising enough. Are you one of those people who eat very little compared to other people in your life, and still the weight hangs on like gum on your shoe? If you said yes, this chapter is for you. It can help you identify what may be going on in your body that keeps you from enjoying the weight-loss success so many other people have benefited from on the Weekend Weight-Loss Diet.

This chapter might seem like a downer after I pumped you up in chapter 1. But the truth is that although the Weekend Weight-Loss Diet works for most people to jump-start their long-term weight-loss goals, there are individuals who have certain health conditions or lifestyle issues that make it very difficult to lose weight. If you are one of those folks, unless the underlying challenge is addressed, you could spend a lifetime pursuing weight loss unsuccessfully. Often when problems are corrected that cause both ill health and weight gain, the weight just melts away naturally. As you heal your body, balance your hormones, detoxify your organs of elimination, identify and eliminate foods that pack on the pounds, and creatively deal with emotional eating, you can achieve and maintain a healthy weight for life.

The late Dr. Robert C. Atkins said that about 20 percent of the people on the Atkins diet didn't lose weight because of a yeast overgrowth known as *Candida albicans*.[1] Candidiasis, as it's also called, is one of the conditions that is covered in this chapter, along with metabolic syndrome, chronic fatigue syndrome, fibromyalgia, low thyroid, sleep disorders, digestive disorders (including irritable bowel syndrome, leaky gut syndrome, Crohn's disease, and colitis), food sensitivities, and stress. I encourage you to read through this chapter even if you don't think anything applies to you. You may be surprised as to what you learn about your body.

1. Metabolic Syndrome

Although Gerald Reaven, MD, professor emeritus at Stanford School of Medicine, first identified metabolic syndrome in 1998, its principal component of obesity was not initially emphasized as it is today. Metabolic syndrome is a combination of obesity, hypercholesterolemia, and hypertension linked by an underlying insulin resistance. Any three of the following traits in an individual signify metabolic syndrome:

- Abdominal obesity: a waist circumference over 102 centimeters (40 inches) in men and over 88 centimeters (35 inches) in women

- High serum triglycerides: 150 mg/dl or above

- Low HDL cholesterol: 40 mg/dl or lower in men and 50 mg/dl or lower in women

- High blood pressure: 130/85 or more
- High blood sugar: a fasting blood glucose of 110 mg/dl or above (some groups say 100 mg/dl)

Metabolic syndrome is also associated with excess insulin secretion. Excessive dietary intake of sugar and refined flour products, lack of exercise, and genetic tendencies contribute to insulin resistance and the other characteristics that lead to metabolic syndrome. Insulin signals the cells to absorb glucose from the bloodstream. The body monitors the food we've digested, our blood sugar levels, and our cell demands; it then should release insulin in the right amounts for our needs. A healthy body is insulin sensitive, not resistant.

Today most of the calories in an average American diet come from carbohydrates, with many of those being simple carbohydrates—sugars in the form of sweets and refined flour—that quickly enter the bloodstream. The body has to release high levels of insulin to keep the level of glucose in the bloodstream from spiraling out of control. Letting your blood sugar get too high is simply not acceptable. The resulting excess of insulin in the bloodstream is called hyperinsulinemia. The body wasn't designed for prolonged high levels of insulin; it disrupts cellular metabolism and spreads inflammation. Over time the cells quit responding to this signal, and the body becomes insulin resistant. It's like knocking on a person's door to the point of annoyance; no one answers.

Insulin resistance causes weight gain because it disrupts fat metabolism. When the cells won't absorb the extra glucose circulating in the bloodstream, the liver converts it into fat. And guess what? Normal fat cells are loaded with glucose receptors that are sensitive to insulin signals. So while the fat cells are gobbling up glucose, the other cells are actually "starved" for glucose. This person feels tired a lot and tends to eat more carbohydrate-rich foods trying to boost energy, which makes her situation even worse. It becomes a frustrating cycle.

The lifestyle changes that turn this syndrome around start with a low-glycemic diet and avoidance of *all* sugar. The Weekend Weight-Loss Diet is an ideal way to start such an eating plan. On this two-day diet the emphasis is on vegetable juices. You should eliminate sugar and even reduce fruit; juice only low-sugar fruit such as a green apple or berries, and lemon and lime. Sweeteners, no matter what we call them, are still sugars. Most natural sweeteners such as honey, agave syrup, and pure maple syrup are a little better than refined sugars, in that they have some nutrients and aren't bleached and refined; however, they are still sugar. (If you do sweeten with honey, I prefer you use raw honey, which is why you'll find this in some of my recipes that you can try when you move beyond the Weekend Weight-Loss Diet.) In addition, you should avoid caffeine and tobacco. Include plenty of healthy fats, especially the omega-3 fats, and avoid animal fats. Limit your salt intake, using only Celtic sea salt, and make sure you exercise during your weekend program and then at least three to four times per week thereafter. All this should help your cells become more responsive to insulin and curb overproduction of insulin. Weight loss should follow without a lot of effort. But the best news is that your health will improve immensely.

2. HYPOTHYROIDISM

People with an underactive thyroid tend to have a very low basal metabolic rate. One of the most noticeable symptoms of low thyroid is weight gain and difficulty losing weight. Sometimes an overactive thyroid can mimic an underactive one by causing weight gain, but this is less common. For people with low thyroid who are dieting, their metabolism continues to slow down as calories are reduced. That's why some people with low thyroid can have weight gain even when they severely restrict their calories.

More women than men suffer from a sluggish thyroid, or hypothyroidism, and many more women than men with thyroid issues have problems with weight gain. Most thyroid problems occur within the gland itself, but it often isn't discovered until other hormonal imbalances develop. Often thyroid issues, menopause, and weight gain appear together.

Thyroid problems develop in women more than men because:

- Often women spend a lot of their lives dieting, usually in a yo-yo pattern of excess eating and strict fasting. This undermines the metabolism and decreases the metabolic rate, a multipart factor impacting the thyroid, especially during perimenopause.

- Women more than men tend to internalize stress, which affects the adrenal and thyroid glands. Overactive adrenal glands produce excess cortisol, which interferes with thyroid hormones and deposits fat around the midsection. In addition, fatigue caused by overstressed adrenals increases cravings for sweets and refined carbohydrates to provide quick energy and feel-good hormones.

- Women's bodies require a delicate balance of hormones such as estrogen and progesterone. These can be upset when the body is stressed, when it is slightly acidic, or when it is not getting enough nutritional support. This results in hormonal imbalances, which act as a trigger for thyroid problems.

There are a number of symptoms that can be experienced when you have an underactive thyroid, such as fatigue, depression, weight gain, cold hands and feet, low body temperature, sensitivity to cold, a feeling of always being chilled, joint pain, headaches, menstrual disorders, insomnia, dry skin, puffy eyes, hair loss, brittle nails, constipation, mental dullness, frequent infections, hoarse voice, ringing in the ears, dizziness, and low sex drive. If you suspect that you have low thyroid, you should get tested. However, be aware that you may not test as hypothyroid, yet you may still have an underactive thyroid gland. (You can take the Thyroid Health Quiz in my book *The Coconut Diet*. I have extensive information on thyroid health in chapter 4 of that book and more than seventy delicious recipes using coconut oil.)

Nourish Your Thyroid

In order to fix your metabolism, you need to nourish your thyroid gland and work on your overall health. Here's what you can do.

- Consume plenty of iodine-rich foods, including fish, seafood, sea vegetables, eggs, cranberries, spinach, and green bell peppers.

- Use Celtic sea salt; avoid iodized sodium chloride (table salt). Celtic sea salt naturally contains iodine with a full complement of minerals that work together.

- Take a good multivitamin-mineral supplement. See Appendix A for recommendations on a good multivitamin.

- Avoid or limit goitrogens, which block iodine absorption by the thyroid gland. The most commonly eaten of these foods are soy and peanuts. Watch out for soybean oil in salad dressings and snack foods; also textured vegetable protein, which is soy. It's used as filler in a lot of snack foods and energy bars. Use almond, oat, or rice milk instead of soy milk. And avoid soy ice cream, soy cheese, and soy protein powder.

- Avoid fluoride. Fluoride will impede the absorption of iodine. Fluoride is added to city water treatment all across America. Unless you have a special water purification system that takes out fluoride, you will be drinking it. It's added to toothpaste, so you will need to shop for fluoride-free toothpaste. And avoid getting your teeth painted with fluoride at the dental office.

- Use virgin coconut oil in food preparation. Poly-unsaturated oils such as soy, corn, safflower, and sunflower oil are damaging to the thyroid gland because they oxidize quickly and become rancid. The opposite effect happens with virgin coconut oil; it does not oxidize and turn rancid easily. For more information, see Appendix A.

3. SLEEP DISORDERS

Have you noticed that when you don't get enough sleep you have the munchies? Could those nights up late at the computer, watching TV, or restlessly tossing in bed be altering your metabolism?

Studies have shown that people who are sleep deprived eat more food, often choosing the most fattening fare. Dr. Robert Stickgold, associate professor of psychiatry and a neuroscientist specializing in sleep research at Harvard, said, "Up at 2:00 a.m., working on a paper, a steak or pasta is not very attractive. You'll grab the candy bar instead. It probably has to do with the glucose regulation going off. It could be that a good chunk of our epidemic of obesity is actually an epidemic of sleep deprivation."[2]

In the last forty years, the rate of obesity in the United States has nearly tripled to one in three adults. But consider this: over the same period, the US population has subtracted, on average, more than an hour from their nightly slumber and about two hours since 1910, when the average person slept 9 hours a night. According to the National Sleep Foundation, people in the United States typically sleep about 6.8 hours on weeknights (that's about 2 hours less than they did a century ago) and 7.4 hours on weekends.[3]

In a study of the sleep habits of 3,682 individuals, conducted by Columbia University, those who slept less than 4 hours a night were

73 percent more likely to be obese than those who slept 7 to 9 hours nightly. Individuals who slept 6 hours a night were 23 percent more likely to be obese. Other studies have reported that sleeping 6.5 or fewer hours for successive nights can cause potentially harmful metabolic, hormonal, and immune changes that can lead to illnesses and diseases such as cancer, diabetes, obesity, and heart disease.[4]

How Sleep Affects Hunger Hormones

There are hormones that make you hungry and hormones that control your appetite. And research shows they are significantly influenced by how much sleep you get. Here's what studies have revealed:

- Five appetite-influencing hormones can get out of whack when you don't get enough sleep, which significantly affects how much you eat.[5]

- When you are sleep deprived, your metabolism can really suffer, which causes weight gain.[6]

- Appetite-suppressing hormones and appetite-stimulating hormones are best regulated when you get seven to nine hours sleep per night.[7]

- You won't crave high-calorie, carbohydrate-rich foods nearly as much when you get adequate, refreshing sleep.[8]

- Sufficient sleep will help you manage your blood sugar more effectively, which helps you manage your appetite. Even one week of sleep deprivation can set off a temporary diabetic effect causing you to crave sugar and other fattening foods.[9]

Never again feel guilty about sleeping. But what if you want to sleep and can't? There's a lot you can do to correct sleep disorders. Get a copy of my book *Sleep Away the Pounds*, where you will find dozens of remedies to help you correct a host of sleep problems.

You can also check out the amino acid program I discovered a number of years ago when I couldn't sleep. (See Appendix A.) I was actually working on my sleep and weight-loss book when I developed horrible insomnia. I had a urinalysis test done, which showed that some of my major brain neurotransmitters were really out of whack, namely serotonin, dopamine, epinephrine, and norepinephrine. I discovered that when they get that far out of balance, it's very hard to bring them back in balance with diet alone. The right amino acids tailored to my specific needs worked amazingly fast. Within about three weeks, I was sleeping deeply again.

The Amino Acid Program Can Help You Sleep

Amino acids can help balance neurotransmitters that influence sleep. Neurotransmitters are the natural chemicals manufactured in the body from the proteins we consume. They facilitate communication throughout the body and brain. Two neurotransmitters play a very significant role in a good sleep cycle—serotonin and norepinephrine. We need enough serotonin to fully convert to melatonin as well as enough norepinephrine.

When we awake in the morning, our excitatory or stimulating neurotransmitters, such as norepinephrine, should be high. The excitatory neurotransmitters need to fall all day long for a good sleep cycle to occur at night. If your serotonin is too low or your norepinephrine is too high (or too low), you will have insomnia. When they're balanced, you should get a good night's sleep, which means eight to nine hours of deep, restful sleep for most people.

Serotonin is converted from the amino acid L-tryptophan, which is broken down into 5-hydroxytryptophan (5-HTP) for the creation of serotonin. The body often needs larger amounts of this amino acid than we get from food. Additionally, other cofactors such as B vitamins and enzymes must be present for this to occur. Since L-tryptophan breaks down into 5-HTP at a very low percentage, often 5-HTP is taken as a supplement. Dosages should be based on testing, however. B vitamins are among the necessary nutrients for the creation and transport of L-tryptophan and conversion of 5-HTP into serotonin. They should also be taken as part of a complete brain wellness plan. Omega-3 fatty acids and varied protein consumption are imperative. You may greatly benefit from an amino acid supplement program tailored to your body's specific needs. (See Appendix A for more information.)

Also, be aware that if the liver is congested, you may have a tough time sleeping. I have noticed amazing improvements in my quality of sleep after I've completed a liver cleanse. Take heart if sleep has been an issue for you. If you can get to the root of the problem, you can correct a sleep disorder by making the necessary changes.

Sleeping in a few extra minutes has its advantages. Research shows that if you increase your sleep by just thirty minutes per night, your chances of losing weight go up exponentially.[10]

It's apparent that getting plenty of refreshing sleep on a consistent basis, and enough sleep to meet your body's needs, could be far better for your weight-loss goals than diet pills and just as important as working out or eating right.

4. Candidiasis

Candida albicans are usually benign yeasts (or fungus) that naturally inhabit the digestive tract. They are meant to live in harmonious relationship with beneficial intestinal flora. In healthy people, they don't present a problem because they're kept in check by the good gut bacteria.

But when the good bacteria are destroyed by the use of antibiotics or other medications, yeasts flourish. Combine that with many of our twenty-first-century lifestyle habits, such as a diet rich in sugar, refined carbohydrates, alcohol, birth control pills, and stress, and the perfect environment is created that encourages yeast growth that's out of control.

Candidiasis can cause a variety of symptoms, such as cravings for sugar, bread, or alcohol; weight gain; fatigue; vaginitis; immune system dysfunction; depression; digestive disorders; frequent ear and sinus infections; intense itching; chemical sensitivities; canker sores; and ringworm. Some people say they feel "sick all over." If you think you may have a yeast overgrowth, you can take the Candida Quiz in my book *The Coconut Diet*.

Conquering yeast: A key for successful weight loss

Focusing on removing yeast from the body rewards you with a feeling of well-being and steady, sustainable, and healthy weight loss. If the yeast is allowed to continue its growth, it can mutate into a fungus that can spread throughout the body. Unless halted, the fungus will not stop; it can completely destroy your health. In worst-case scenarios, the sufferer may become bedridden because the *C. albicans* fungus can completely drain a healthy body of all energy by pumping it full of toxins (mycotoxins).

Americans have embraced the low-carbohydrate diet for its ability to reduce their waist size when other diets have failed. But an equally important benefit of a low-carbohydrate diet is that it starves yeast of their primary food—sugars. A person with systemic *C. albicans* will often crave sugar and simple carbohydrates because this is the main source of nutrients for yeast. Mood swings, PMS, and depression are associated with the rapid change in blood sugar levels caused by yeast. People complain of gas and bloating that yeast causes by fermenting foods in their intestines. This naturally releases gas just as champagne and beer do. Yeasts also produce alcohol via fermentation, which is absorbed through the gut and may cause symptoms of brain fog, altered behavior, and difficulty concentrating.

Chlorophyll deactivates systemic yeast

Molds, fungus, and yeasts (all fungi) are single or multicell organisms that can cause us to gain weight. Yeast cells numbering in the millions can colonize the digestive track. Those who have accumulated higher than normal levels usually will crave carbs—sweets, alcohol, and starches such as bread, potatoes, white rice, crackers, rolls, bagels, pasta, and pizza because the yeasts demand to be fed. And those cravings are often uncontrollable. Eating this stuff leads to bloating and weight gain. A person may also lose muscle strength. If they continue to feed the fungi by eating simple carbohydrates and starches, the whole situation becomes a no-win frustrating cycle—the strength of the fungi increases. More fat is produced. And many health problems worsen.

C. albicans produce a large number of biologically active substances called mycotoxins, which are highly acidic waste products. These toxins are secreted to serve the fungi by protecting it against viruses, bacteria, and parasites. They can get into the bloodstream and produce an array of central nervous system symptoms such as fatigue, confusion, irritability, mental fogginess, memory loss, depression, dizziness, mood swings, headache, nausea, numbness, and hypoglycemia. And these toxins can produce chronic illness, frequently described as "feeling sick all over."

The body has difficulty cleansing fungi spores from the mucous membranes throughout the body and controlling its overgrowth systemically. One of the actions of mucus is to collect and absorb harmful microbes like toxic fungi. An overgrowth can contribute to illnesses like sinusitis and congestion. Under normal conditions these organisms can be controlled, but when the amount coming in or reproducing exceeds the body's systems of control, the accumulations create problems.

Research at Oregon State University has shown that chlorophyll binds to mycotoxins, thus blocking them from entering the bloodstream.[11] This makes the beautiful green juice recipes in chapter 7 potentially life-changing for up to 80 million Americans (70 percent of them women) who suffer with an overgrowth of *C. albicans*.[12]

Green juices and savory green smoothies can make a big difference for you if you suffer with symptoms such as chronic fatigue, persistent sinusitis, allergies, carb cravings, and vaginal infections related to yeast overgrowth. The fungi do not like an environment rich in chlorophyll, which is a compound found in plants that is essential to photosynthesis and gives plants their color. Foods rich in chlorophyll make the fungi's job much tougher. It is very alkaline and neutralizes the acidity produced by the mycotoxins. It also binds them, stopping the fungi's destructive cycle. So pour yourself a big glass of green juice and knock the fungi out!

Probiotics: Weight-loss heroes

The composition of microflora, the bacteria in the digestive tract, could help to determine how many calories are absorbed from food. Recent research suggests that these good bacteria can increase metabolism and weight loss. *Nature* reported that overweight people have different microorganisms in the gut than lean people, suggesting that obesity may have a microbial aspect to it. According to the report, when an obese person loses weight, their microbial population reverts back to that of a lean person.[13]

Japanese scientists also discovered that probiotics promoted weight loss. They recruited eighty-seven overweight people who were given 200 grams of fermented milk every day for twelve weeks. The participants were randomly divided into two groups: those whose fermented milk contained *Lactobacillus gasseri* (a probiotic) and those whose fermented milk did not. Significant decreases in body weight, BMI, waist circumference, and hips were observed in the Lactobacillus group but not in the control group.[14]

Probiotics are dietary supplements or foods that contain the kind of good bacteria naturally found in the body. According to Mayo Clinic nutritionist Katherine Zeratsky, "These microorganisms may help with digestion and offer protection from harmful bacteria, just as the existing 'good' bacteria in your body do."[15]

Most people think of yogurt when they consider foods rich in probiotics. But raw vegetables, fresh veggie juice, and fermented foods such as miso and sauerkraut add plenty of good "living" bacteria to the intestinal tract. Keep in mind that cooking kills them. This is another reason why people on a living foods diet often lose weight.

Two Super Foods That Kill Yeast

There are several foods that will help to lower your yeast levels and get you on track to controlling them. Include plenty of the following foods:

1. *Raw garlic.* Two antifungal actions of raw garlic (cooked doesn't work) have been identified by studies at Putra University in Malaysia: it stops the formation of *hyphae*—long strands that branch off of yeast and enable it to spread, and it causes yeast cells to die prematurely.[16] You need to eat at least one raw clove a day—or juice it with one of the recipes in chapter 7.

2. *Organic virgin coconut oil.* A study in 2007 in the Department of Medical Microbiology and Parasitology at University College Hospital in Nigeria demonstrated the effectiveness of virgin coconut oil as an antifungal agent that killed *C. albicans.* Researchers concluded that coconut oil destroyed 100 percent of the yeast cells on contact. Specifically, credit goes to lauric, caprylic, and capric acids in coconut oil that worked synergistically to split open the protective outer wall

of yeast cells. The dose used was 3 tablespoons daily.[17] Coconut oil can be substituted in place of other dietary fats such as butter or oils.

Numerous animal and human research studies have confirmed that replacing long-chain fatty acids—found in polyunsaturated oils such as corn, safflower, sunflower, and soy oil—with medium-chain fatty acids (MCFAs)—found in coconut oil—results in both decreased body weight and reduced fat deposits. This is because MCFAs are easily digested and turned into energy, and they stimulate metabolism. Several studies have also shown that MCFAs can enhance athletic performance.[18]

Another benefit of coconut oil is that it boosts the thyroid gland, helps your body's immune system to function better, and aids in weight loss.[19]

5. DIGESTIVE DISORDERS

The major function of the digestive system is to break down and absorb nutrients. When your gastrointestinal system isn't functioning up to par, essential nutrients that are necessary to maintain proper weight and good health may not be absorbed adequately from the foods we eat, even if we are eating a healthy diet. This can lead to nutrient deficiencies, cravings, overeating, weight gain, and poor health.

When you're eating a whole-foods diet and avoiding sugar and other refined carbohydrates, you should not gain weight. However, many people who have switched over to a healthy diet and have even greatly limited their carbohydrate intake still have problems losing weight. You may be one who suffers from poor digestion and experiences symptoms such as gas, belching, constipation, or a digestive disorder that prevents you from properly breaking down and utilizing your food. You can have the best nutrition on Earth, and it will go to waste unless you are able to digest it well.

When the body suffers from a digestive disorder, it becomes difficult to digest fats. So while it's important to eliminate unhealthy fats from our diet and switch to healthy fats such as fish oil, virgin coconut oil, and extra-virgin olive oil, you also need to make sure your digestive system can properly digest the fats you eat. Those with a poorly functioning pancreas have great difficulties in digesting fats. The pancreas produces enzymes that are required for breakdown and absorption of food. For example, lipase, along with bile, functions in the breakdown of fats. Malabsorption (poor absorption) of fat and fat-soluble vitamins occurs when there is a deficiency of lipase.

The digestive system is interrelated, and one poorly functioning aspect of the system usually affects all the others. For example, the liver manufactures bile, which is important in the absorption of fats, oils, and fat-soluble vitamins. When liver function is impaired and there is not enough bile produced, stools can become quite hard and difficult to pass. This affects the health of the colon and increases the absorption of toxins from the stool back into the system. Also, bile serves to keep the small intestine free from microorganisms such as *Candida albicans*, which we looked at previously.

Other digestive disorders include indigestion, irritable bowel syndrome (IBS), gastritis, diverticular disease, dysbiosis (altered bacterial flora), and constipation. More severe digestive disorders are known as inflammatory bowel disease (IBD) and include Crohn's disease and ulcerative colitis, characterized by an inflammatory reaction throughout the bowel. IBD sufferers usually experience bouts of diarrhea, cramping, and weight loss.

Simple Steps to Improve Digestion

Whether or not you have been diagnosed with a digestive disorder, if you have trouble with digestion in any form—burping, bloating, and flatulence to more severe problems such as those mentioned above—chances are that your organs of elimination need detoxifying and your digestive system needs some help. This is especially true as you age. There are a number of steps you can take to improve your digestion.

- *Chew your food very well.* Thoroughly chew each bite of food. Carbohydrate digestion begins in the mouth—chewing food thoroughly allows amylase, the digestive enzyme present in saliva, to digest the carbohydrates.

- *Drink enough water every day; that's about eight glasses.* Not drinking enough water is a primary cause of constipation, which promotes an imbalance in bacteria, contributes to inflammation of the intestinal lining, and can even lead to the absorption of larger molecules, a condition known as intestinal permeability.

- *Boost your intake of vitamin C and magnesium.* Deficiencies in these two nutrients can contribute to constipation. Take vitamin C to bowel tolerance (loose stool), and then cut back by about 500 milligrams. This should indicate the amount of vitamin C your body needs. And take magnesium citrate to help improve bowel function. (See Appendix A for more information.)

- *Eat plenty of fiber.* Aim for five to nine servings of vegetables a day. Make some of those vegetables the high-fiber cruciferous veggies such as cauliflower, kale, broccoli, and brussels sprouts. Eat a low-sugar green apple for a snack. Sprinkle ground flaxseeds on your oatmeal or in your morning juice or smoothie. Take products with inulin; it's a prebiotic that is good for the colon. (Inulin is a soluble plant fiber that has a slightly sweet taste.)

- *Deal with food sensitivities.* Food sensitivities are behind many digestive disorders. For example, between one-third and two-thirds of IBS patients report having one or more food intolerances, resulting in bloating, gas, and pain. The most common culprits are dairy, grains, corn, and soy.

- *Boost good gut bacteria (probiotics).* Lactobacillus acidophilus and Bifidobacterium bifidum are considered good probiotic bacteria because they can help to maintain intestinal health.

- *Take supplements that restore digestive health.* Enteric-coated peppermint oil can reduce abdominal pain, bloating, and gas. Digestive enzymes will support the body's own digestive enzymes and aid digestion.

6. FIBROMYALGIA AND FATIGUE

Chronic fatigue syndrome (CFS) is a disabling illness that causes extreme exhaustion, muscle pain, sleep disturbances, cognitive difficulties, and hormonal deficiencies and imbalances. Fibromyalgia is a chronic disorder that causes widespread muscle pain, fatigue, sleep disturbances, cognitive difficulties ("Fibro Fog"), stiffness, and headaches. People with these conditions gain weight due to hormonal imbalances, sleep disturbances, and changes in activity levels. Hormonal imbalances, particularly the hypothyroidism found in CFS patients, cause the metabolism to slow down, leading to weight gain. Cortisol, the "stress hormone," is often low during the day but can also start pumping out during the night, causing sleep problems in CFS patients, and this can contribute to weight gain. Cortisol causes weight gain especially around the waist and stomach.

Improving Fibromyalgia and CFS

To improve these conditions, try the following:

- *Support your adrenal glands.* Most people with fibromyalgia or chronic fatigue syndrome have exhausted adrenal glands. It's important to avoid substances that tax the adrenals, such as caffeine (coffee, black tea, chocolate), soda, alcohol, and sugar; and to include supplements that support the adrenals, such as vitamin C, vitamin B_5, enzymes, and pantothenic acid.

- *Eat a low-glycemic diet.* The Weekend Weight-Loss Diet is ideal for fibromyalgia and CFS sufferers since it is low-glycemic and loaded with nutrients that help the body heal. High-carbohydrate foods should be completely avoided and replaced with vegetables and healthy fats such as avocado, extra-virgin olive oil, and virgin coconut oil.

- *Include foods that are rich in magnesium.* To avoid the low magnesium levels common among CFS and fibromyalgia sufferers, consume magnesium-rich foods such as legumes, seeds, nuts, and green leafy vegetables, especially beet greens, spinach, Swiss chard, collard greens, and parsley. You may also benefit from a supplement combo of magnesium and malic acid. (See Appendix A.)

- *Cleanse your body of toxins.* Cleansing is a very important part of correcting these conditions. I recommend that if you suffer from either CFS or fibromyalgia, you start a cleansing program as soon as possible. (See Appendix A for cleanse program recommendations.)

- *Take 2 to 3 tablespoons of virgin coconut oil each day.* I have received reports from fibromyalgia sufferers who have recovered from this terrible disease and are living pain free after

starting on the coconut diet and the addition of
fresh juice. (See my book *The Coconut Diet.*)

7. Toxic Overload

Many people who struggle with being overweight blame themselves for
lack of discipline or willpower, but environmental health specialists
explain that chemicals in pesticides, plastics, cosmetics, cleaning
solvents, and many other commonly used products build up to
toxic levels in our bodies and break down our natural defenses and
weight-control mechanisms. These foreign substances accumulate
in fat cells because that's the safest place for the body to store them.
The more chemicals and toxins, the more fat the body holds on to; it
will even manufacture more fat cells for storage of these damaging
substances, if needed.

Once toxic material such as organophosphates (a compound
containing phosphate groups) gets into your body, chances are they
will proceed to damage your weight-control systems, making it
harder to lose weight in the future. Synthetic chemicals, which have
been used to fatten up animals for meat production by reducing
their ability to use their own existing fat stores, also contribute to
weight gain in humans. Animals fed low doses of organophosphates
gain weight on less food. While their use as growth promoters
in meat production has been banned after research found them
highly toxic, organophosphates remain a common pesticide. They
are also used in the manufacture of gasoline additives, lubricating
oil, and rubber. This is just one example of the many toxins in our
environment that can disrupt our weight-control systems.

The Weekend Weight-Loss Diet is loaded with antioxidants in
the juices that help detoxify the body and flip the switch from the
weight-gain mode to the weight-loss mode.

Getting rid of toxins and boosting your detoxification system is an essential component of long-term weight control and a healthy metabolism. I have an excellent detoxification program in my books *Juicing, Fasting, and Detoxing for Life* and *The Juice Lady's Guide to Juicing for Health* that will lead you step by step in detoxifying your colon, liver, gallbladder, and kidneys. (See Appendix A for recommendations of cleanse products.)

8. FOOD SENSITIVITY

Reactions to foods are not always immediate. They can occur many hours after eating with symptoms such as bloating and swelling in the hands, feet, ankles, face, abdomen, chin, and around the eyes. It can also account for bags and dark circles under the eyes. Much of the weight gained is fluid retention caused by inflammation and the release of certain hormones. In addition, there is fermentation of foods, particularly carbohydrates, in the intestines, which can result in a swollen, distended belly due to gas.

Symptoms of food sensitivity can include headache, migraine, indigestion or heartburn, fatigue, depression, joint pain or arthritis, canker sores, chronic respiratory symptoms such as wheezing, sinus congestion or bronchitis, and chronic bowel problems such as diarrhea or constipation. The most common food allergens are wheat or gluten, corn, dairy, soy, and sugar. Juicing is very helpful because the food is broken down into a very easily absorbed form that does not cause allergic reactions.

9. STRESS

There are entire books written about the health problems caused by our overstressed modern lifestyles. Stress can cause you to gain weight, whereas relaxing can make you thin. Under any physical or psychological stress, the body is designed to protect itself. It stores calories and conserves weight. It pumps hormones like cortisol into your system, which increase blood fats, sugar, and insulin to prepare the body for "fight or flight."

It is well known that the excess cortisol released during stressful times causes fat to be deposited in the midsection. Without eating more or exercising less, stress alone will cause weight gain and can lead to diabetes. Active relaxation helps to reduce stress, along with inflammation, and to increase fat burning to better control blood sugar. Juicing can help your body deal with stress because it contains many nutrients that feed your body super nutrition. This helps your body deal with stress more effectively.

10. Liver or Gallbladder Congestion

If you reach a plateau at any time during your weight-loss program or you want to accelerate your weight loss and healthy lifestyle plan, you can cleanse your body, starting with the Weekend Weight-Loss Diet. For further cleansing, I also recommend a colon cleanse program and then the seven-day Liver and Gallbladder Cleanse, which are outlined in detail in my books *Juicing, Fasting, and Detoxing for Life* and *The Juice Lady's Guide to Juicing for Health*. A congested liver and gallbladder could prevent you from losing weight. Also, you may find it impossible to shed pounds until you cleanse toxins from your body, especially the organs of elimination.

Chapter 3

Why a Liquid Diet
Jump-Starts Weight Loss

IT MAY SURPRISE you to learn that vegetable juice is the secret ingredient to your weight-loss success. It assists you in becoming slim and healthy due to its alkalinizing, nutrition-packed, energizing properties. Let's face it—juicing is a lot easier than spending all your time chowing down on brussels sprouts, carrots, and broccoli. Don't get me wrong. I recommend that you eat these vegetables often, but really, just how many vegetables can you eat in a day? But you can juice them and drink them with ease.

Because vegetable juice has very little sugar, while offering an abundance of vitamins, minerals, enzymes, and phytonutrients, it's incredibly helpful for weight loss. It offers what your body needs to fight cravings and do its work to keep you healthy. You will not only want to eat fewer calories when you include vegetable juicing in your daily routine, but you will also gain energy. On the other hand, you can eat a whole bag of chips and still want something more to eat because your body was given a lot of empty calories that made you feel sluggish and tired. The biggest plus of a juicing program is that it adds valuable nutrients (vitamins, minerals, enzymes, and phytonutrients) that are easy for your body to absorb and that have a heap of health benefits at minimal calorie cost.

Research Proves the Juice Diet Works!

Two university studies have shown that one to two glasses of vegetable juice a day promote four times the weight loss of non-juice drinkers on the same American Heart Association diet. Both studies were randomized controlled trials, each lasting twelve weeks.[1]

In the study conducted by University of California–Davis among ninety healthy adults between the ages of forty and sixty-five, it was found that each person who drank at least 2 cups of vegetable juice a day met their weight-loss goal while only 7 percent of the non-juice drinkers met it. Participants who drank either 1 or 2 cups of vegetable juice per day lost an average of 4 pounds, while those who drank no vegetable juice lost only 1 pound. The researchers also found that people in the vegetable juice groups had significantly higher vitamin C and potassium intake and a significantly lower intake of carbohydrates. Participants with borderline high blood pressure who drank 1 or 2 cups of vegetable juice lowered their blood pressure significantly.[2]

The vegetable juice drinkers said they enjoyed the juice and felt like they were doing something good for themselves by drinking it. According to Carl Keen, PhD, professor of Nutrition and Internal Medicine at UC–Davis and coauthor of the study, "Enjoyment is so critical to developing good eating habits you can stick with for a long time….Vegetable juice is something that people enjoy, plus it's convenient and portable, which makes it simple to drink every day."[3]

The Baylor College of Medicine study involved eighty-one adults who drank 8 to 16 ounces of vegetable juice daily as part of a calorie-controlled, heart-healthy diet. They showed an average of 4 pounds lost over a twelve-week study period compared with those who did not drink juice and lost only 1 pound. Of the participants in the study, almost three-quarters of whom were women, 83 percent had metabolic syndrome, which is a cluster of risk factors including excess body fat around the midsection, high blood pressure, high blood sugar, and elevated cholesterol.[4]

It is estimated that 47 million Americans have some combination of these risk factors, placing them at increased risk for diabetes and heart disease.[5] That's why the low-glycemic Weekend Weight-Loss Diet works so well for weight loss and can be especially helpful for people with blood sugar challenges such as those with metabolic syndrome. (You'll learn more about metabolic syndrome in the next chapter.)

The Baylor College of Medicine study mentioned earlier involved a large percentage of participants with metabolic syndrome—a cluster of characteristics that include weight gain at the midsection, insulin resistance, low HDL, high blood pressure, and elevated triglycerides. If not corrected by following a low-glycemic diet, this syndrome usually evolves into diabetes. Most of the people with metabolic syndrome in the study lost weight when adding vegetable juice to their diet, four times the weight of others that did not drink juice.

Most of us are very aware of the side effects of unhealthy appetite suppressants or risky surgery, but sometimes people feel that they have no other option. I'm here to tell you that you *do* have options, and the Weekend Weight-Loss Diet is one of the healthiest options on Earth! The vegetable juices act as healthy, harmless appetite suppressants. You can opt for a glass of fresh veggie juice before your main meal and quickly experience those hunger pangs taking an exit. That's just one of the secret reasons why the Weekend Weight-Loss Diet works.

Vegetable juice can also play an important role in stabilizing blood sugar, a vital factor in appetite control, because it's very low in sugar. Now that's something to get excited about. Sugar and foods like refined flour products (such as bread, rolls, and pasta) that quickly turn into sugar in your body cause spikes and dips in blood sugar. When your blood sugar gets low, you can get ravenously hungry and sometimes grouchy. The sugar percentage of vegetable juice is much lower than that of fruit juice and the calorie count is up to 50 percent less, yet the juice succeeds in satisfying a sweet tooth. Amazing! This makes juicing an absolute must for successful dieting. Experiment with carrot; greens such as kale, chard, or collards; lemon; and ginger, or a combination of carrot, Jerusalem artichoke, lemon, and parsley juice when a carb craving hits. The juice jolt will give those cravings a knockout!

When you satisfy your body with alkaline-rich, nutrient-dense juices and foods and your blood sugar stabilizes, your appetite for junk food, sweets, and high-carb fare begins to fade away. You may notice that your fatigue vanishes and energy zooms. You will feel more like getting up and going in the morning, working out, and getting things done. Like so many other juicing enthusiasts, you may also notice that your focus improves dramatically. That's because your brain is being well fed. When you eat nutrient-depleted food, your brain doesn't get as much of the raw materials it needs to make reactions happen. Things misfire, and you walk around looking for your car keys for ten minutes when they're in your pocket all the time. Now you can say good-bye to brain fog!

Seven Ways Juicing Helps You Lose Weight

I've been talking since the beginning of this book about all of the health benefits of the juices I recommend in the Weekend Weight-Loss Diet. But in case you're like me and it helps you to see things at a glance, here is a quick list of seven ways juicing helps people lose weight.

1. It supplies an abundance of nutrients that satisfy the body. Cravings usually diminish quickly.

2. It feeds the brain supernutrients that send a signal to the body that it's satisfied. People often say they aren't hungry after a big glass of fresh veggie juice.

3. Live juices detoxify the body. Toxins can actually cause us to gain weight. It's true. And they can make it very difficult to lose fat.

4. A juice diet is energizing. For a majority of people, fatigue vanishes and workouts get easier. When you work out, you build muscle and burn calories. The more muscle you develop, the more calories you burn, even when resting.

5. It's low in calories. If you're counting them, this program is low in those little energy units that push up the numbers on the bathroom scale.

6. It is low glycemic, meaning it's devoid of fattening carbs.

7. It's a high-alkaline diet. This is a major factor to consider. Actually, the body stores acids in fat cells to protect delicate tissues and organs, making it tough to get rid of fat when the diet is predominantly acidic. Listen up—the body will actually make fat to store acids when it runs out of storage space. When you achieve a healthy pH balance, your body can start letting go of fat cells.

SEVEN VEGETABLE AND FRUIT JUICES THAT HELP PROMOTE WEIGHT LOSS

Let's take a look at seven juices that have the biggest affect on your weight-loss goals.

1. Asparagus juice. Asparagus juice is a natural diuretic. It contains asparagine—a crystalline amino acid that boosts kidney performance, thereby improving waste removal from the body. You can juice the stems that you would normally throw away, which is good conservation of produce.

2. Beet juice. Beets are a natural diuretic that are also thought to help break up fatty deposits.

3. Cabbage juice. Cabbage is thought to aid in breakdown of fatty deposits, especially around the abdominal region.

4. Celery juice. Celery juice is a diuretic and has calming properties. Celery is also good source of natural sodium.

5. Cranberry juice. Cranberries are a diuretic. Juice up cranberries with lemon and a low-sugar green apple; it tastes like lemonade and makes a delicious weight-loss treat.

6. Cucumber juice. Cucumbers help increase urination and aid in flushing out toxins. Cucumbers are rich in sulfur and silicon, which stimulate the kidneys to better remove uric acid. The silicon is also great for hair and nails and helps to prevent hair loss and nail splitting.

7. Tomato juice. Tomatoes contain citric acid and malic acid, which enhance the body's metabolism, promoting more efficient calorie burning.

Drinking a glass of vegetable juice before each meal can help curb your appetite. If you choose the ingredients with some care, you can get a double dividend of appetite control. The best vegetables to use when juicing for weight loss are *negative calorie foods*—those that require more calories to digest than they contain. Include more negative calorie foods such as dark greens, broccoli, carrots, Jerusalem artichoke, fennel, and cabbage, which are among the best vegetables to use in juice recipes for weight loss. Also consider using asparagus, cucumber, and celery, which are natural diuretics that can alleviate water retention.

In addition, carrot juice diluted with cucumber and greens such as kale, chard, collards, or parsley can help to maintain blood sugar levels, which will help prevent hunger. Since carrot juice is sweet, it can also help to satisfy sugar cravings, but due to its higher sugar content, it should be diluted with low-sugar green veggies. Another vegetable to try for curing a sweet tooth is Jerusalem artichoke. However, although it reduces sugar cravings, Jerusalem artichoke is bland, so it's best combined with things such as carrot, cucumber, and lemon juice to bring out its flavor.

Frequently Asked Questions

Now that you know in theory just how effective juicing is for weight loss, you will want to experience it firsthand. In this chapter, I'll help you get started on this weekend program with some guidelines for juicing and choosing a good juicer. But first, here are answers to some frequently asked questions along with plenty of tips to make this a very easy plan to follow.

Why not just eat the fruits and vegetables instead of juicing them?

Always eat your vegetables and fruit. But juice them too! There are at least three reasons why juicing should be included in your lifestyle.

1. You can juice far more produce than you would probably eat in a day. It takes a long time to chew raw veggies. Chewing is a very good thing. It's important for your jaw muscles and your teeth. However, there's only so much time in a day that most of us have for chewing up raw foods. We are no longer hunters and gatherers. One day I timed how long it would take for me to eat five medium-size carrots. (That's what I often juice for my husband and me, along with cucumber;

lemon; ginger root; beet; greens such as kale, chard, or collards; and celery.) It took me about fifty minutes to eat them. Not only do I not have that kind of time every day, but also my jaw was so tired afterward that I could hardly move it.

2. You can juice parts of the plant you would not usually eat, such as beet stems and leaves, celery leaves, the white pithy part of the lemon with the seeds, asparagus stems, kohlrabi leaves, broccoli stems, and kale ribs. Not only is that good nutrition, but it is also good economy.

3. Juice is broken down so well that it's very easy to digest. It also spares digestion, meaning that the organs that produce enzymes don't have to work as hard. It is estimated that juice is at work in the system in about twenty to thirty minutes. And, regarding ailments, juice is therapy for this very reason. When the body has to work hard to break down veggies, for example, it can spend a lot of energy on the digestive process. Juicing does the work for you. So when you drink a glass of fresh vegetable juice, all those life-giving nutrients go to work right away to heal and repair your body, giving it energy for its work of rejuvenation.

Don't we need the fiber that's lost in juicing?

It's true that we need to eat whole vegetables, fruit, sprouts, legumes, and whole grains for fiber. We drink juice for the extra nutrients; it's better than any vitamin pill. And regarding weight loss, we drink vegetable juices for appetite control. I also recommend juice as therapy in my book for more than fifty ailments: *The Juice Lady's Guide to Juicing for Health.*

Whole fruits and vegetables have insoluble and soluble fiber. Both types of fiber are very important for colon health. The insoluble fiber is lost when you juice; however, soluble fiber is present in juice in the form of gums and pectins. Pectins are especially high in lemons and limes. Soluble fiber is excellent for the digestive tract. It also helps to lower blood cholesterol, stabilize blood sugar, and improve good bowel bacteria.

Are a lot of nutrients lost with the fiber?

In the past, some people thought that a significant amount of nutrients remained with the fiber after juicing, but that theory has been disproved. The US Department of Agriculture (USDA) analyzed twelve fruits and found that 90 percent of the antioxidant nutrients they measured was in the juice rather than the fiber. That is why fresh juice makes such a great supplement in the diet.

Is fresh juice better than commercially processed juice?

Fresh juice is "live food" packed with vitamins and enzymes. These nutrients are destroyed with heat. That's why I consider bottled juice dead food. Fresh juice also contains that living ingredient, known as biophotons (light energy), that revitalizes the body and even nourishes the DNA.

In contrast, commercially processed canned, bottled, frozen, or packaged juices have been pasteurized, which means the juice has been heated, and many of the "living nutrients"—vitamins, enzymes, and light energy—are virtually gone. You're left with primarily sugar and water. When people say they think juice is high in sugar, they're right if they are talking about bottled fruit juice.

You'll also be getting a wider variety of vegetables and fruit if you make your own juice and choose veggies such as kale, beets with leaves and stems, kohlrabi with leaves, collard greens, Swiss chard, arugula, rapini, and mustard greens. These ingredients would rarely go into commercial juice. My recipes include all these veggies, plus Jerusalem artichokes, jícama, green cabbage, ginger, celery leaves, black dino kale, and parsley. These sweet, crisp tubers and healthy greens are not found in any processed juices I've seen.

How much produce does it take to make a glass of juice?

People often wonder if it takes a bushel basket of produce to make a glass of juice and if they'll go broke in the process. Actually, if you're using a good juicer, it takes a surprisingly small amount of produce. For example, all of the following items yield about one 8-ounce glass of juice: one large apple, one large cucumber, or five to seven carrots. The following each yield about 4 ounces of juice: three large (13-inch) stalks of celery or one medium tomato. The key is to get a good juicer that yields a dry pulp. I've used juicers that ejected very wet pulp. When I ran the pulp through the juicer again, I got a lot of juice and the pulp was still wet. If the rpm is too high or the juicer is not efficient in other ways, you'll waste a lot of produce, and it will cost a lot of money.

Will juicing cost a lot of money?

You can figure the cost of a glass of juice is less than a latte. With three or four carrots, half a lemon, a chunk of ginger root, a stalk of celery, half a cucumber, and a fistful of leafy greens, you will probably spend about two to three dollars, depending on the season, the area of the country, and the store.

A new study just released by the USDA Economic Research Service shows just how affordable fruits and vegetables really are. Getting the recommended amount costs only $2 to $2.50 per day. Researchers also found no significant difference between the average prices of fresh and processed fruits and vegetables.[6]

But wait—there are also hidden savings. You may not need as many vitamin supplements. What's that worth? And you'll probably need far less over-the-counter medications such as painkillers, sleeping aids, antacids, and cold, cough, and flu medicines. And then there's time not lost from work. What happens when you run out of sick days? Or if you're self-employed, you've missed out on income each day you're sick. With the immune-building, disease-fighting properties of fresh juice, you should stay well. That's a whopping savings!

Should diabetics juice?

I've often heard people say they can't juice because they have diabetes. You can juice vegetables if you have sugar metabolism problems, but you should choose low-sugar veggies and only low-sugar fruit such as lemons and limes. Carrots and beets would be too high in sugar. You could add one or two carrots to a juice recipe or a very small beet or part of a beet, but they should be diluted with cucumber juice and dark leafy greens. You may use lemon and lime, but other fruits are higher in sugar and should be avoided. Berries are low in sugar, especially cranberries, and can be added to juice recipes. Green apples are lower in sugar than yellow or red apples. But I'd don't recommend that you use apples. Keep your juices very low in sugar.

I've worked with people who have reversed their type 2 diabetes by juicing low-sugar vegetables and eating many more living foods, along with a low-glycemic diet. However, your doctor or health care professional will know your personal situation, so make sure you schedule a call or visit to discuss these options before changing your diet.

How to Choose the Right Juicer

Choosing a juicer that is right for you can make the difference between juicing daily and never juicing again, so it's important to get one that works well for your lifestyle.

People often ask me if they can use their blender as a juicer. You can't use a blender to make juice. A juicer separates the liquid from the pulp (insoluble fiber). A blender combines or liquefies everything that is placed in it; it doesn't separate the insoluble fiber from the juice. If you think it might be a good idea to have all that insoluble fiber like carrot, beet, or celery pulp in your juice for added fiber, I can tell you from experience that it tastes like juicy sawdust. For the clear juice, which is juice you'll enjoy and drink every day, you need a good juicer. Look for the following features:

- *Adequate horsepower (hp).* Look for a juicer with 0.3 to 1.0 hp. Weak-motored machines with low horsepower ratings must run at extremely high rpm (revolutions per minute). A machine's rpm does not accurately reflect its ability to perform effectively because rpm is calculated when the juicer is running idle, not while it is juicing. When you feed produce into a low-power machine, the rpm will be reduced dramatically, and sometimes the juicer will come to a full stop. I have "killed" some machines on the first carrot I juiced.

- *Efficient at extracting juice.* I've used a number of juicers that wasted a lot of produce; there was considerable juice left in the pulp. You should not be able to squeeze juice out of the leftover pulp. Some machines are not efficient, even some expensive ones I've tried, and the pulp comes out wet. I've had people tell me they were spending a lot of money on produce. It often turned out that they had an inefficient juicer.

- *Sustained blade speed during juicing.* Look for a machine that has electronic circuitry that sustains blade speed during juicing.

- *Able to juice all types of produce.* Make sure the machine can juice tough, hard vegetables, such as carrots and beets, as well as delicate greens, such as parsley, lettuce, and herbs. Make sure it doesn't need a special citrus attachment. For wheatgrass juice, you'll need a wheatgrass juicer or a juicer that presses the juice, such as a single or double auger or twin-gear machine, also known as a masticating juicer. Be aware that the machines that juice wheatgrass along with other vegetables and fruit take more time to use. They usually have a smaller mouth, so you have to cut produce up into smaller pieces. Some are more time consuming to clean as well.

- *Large feed tube.* Look for a large feed tube if you don't have a lot of time to devote to juicing. Cutting your produce into small pieces before juicing takes extra time.

- *Ejects pulp.* Choose a juicer that ejects pulp into a receptacle. This design is far better than one in which all the pulp stays inside the machine and has to be scooped out frequently. Juicers that keep the pulp in the center basket rather than ejecting it cannot juice continuously. You'll need to stop the machine often to wash it out. Plus, you can line the pulp catcher with a free plastic baggie from the grocery store produce section, and you won't have to wash the receptacle each time. When you're finished juicing, you can either toss the baggie with the pulp or use it in cooking or composting, but you won't need to wash this part of the juicer.

- *Only a few parts to clean.* Look for a juicer with only a few parts to clean that are also dishwasher safe. The more parts a juicer has and the more complicated the parts are to wash, the longer it will take to clean up and the more time it will take to put it back together. That makes it less likely you will use your machine daily. I just rinse my juicer parts and let them air dry. (For juicer recommendations, see Appendix A.)

How to Get the Most From Juicing

Juicing is a very simple process. Simple as the procedure is, though, it helps to keep a few guidelines in mind to get the best results.

- *Wash all produce before juicing.* Fruit and vegetable washes are available at many grocery and health food stores. They wash away surface dirt and mold and help to eliminate surface pesticides, but they don't get rid of pesticides in the water and fiber of the plant. Cut away all moldy, bruised, or damaged areas of the produce.

- *Always peel oranges, tangerines, tangelos, and grapefruit* before juicing because the skins of these citrus fruit contain volatile oils that can cause digestive problems like a stomachache. Lemon and lime peels can be juiced, if organic, but they do add a distinct flavor that is not one of my favorites for most recipes. I usually peel them. Leave as much of the white pithy part on the citrus fruit as possible, since it contains the most vitamin C and bioflavonoids, which together create the best uptake for your immune cells. Always peel mangoes and papayas, since their skins contain an irritant that is harmful when eaten in quantity.

  Also, peel all produce that is not labeled organic, even though the largest concentration of nutrients is in and next to the skin. For example, nonorganic cucumbers are often waxed, trapping pesticides. You don't want the wax or the pesticides in your juice. The peels and skins of sprayed fruits and vegetables contain the largest concentration of pesticides.

- *Remove pits, stones, and hard seeds* from such fruits as peaches, plums, apricots, cherries, and mangoes. Softer seeds from cucumbers, oranges, lemons, limes, watermelons, cantaloupes, grapes, and apples can be juiced without a problem. Because of their chemical composition, large quantities of apple seeds should not be juiced for young children under the age of two, but they should not cause problems for older children and adults.

- *You can juice the stems and leaves* of most produce such as beet stems and leaves, strawberry caps, celery leaves, broccoli stems, and small grape stems—they offer nutrients too. Discard larger grape stems, as they can dull the juicer blade. Also remove carrot and rhubarb greens because they contain toxic substances. Cut off the ends of carrots since this is the part that molds first.

- *Cut fruits and vegetables into sections or chunks* that will fit your juicer's feed tube. You'll learn from experience what can be added whole or what size works best for your machine. If you have a large feed tube, you won't have to cut up very much.

- *Some fruits and vegetables don't juice well.* Most produce contains a lot of water, which is ideal for juicing. The vegetables and fruits that contain less water, such as bananas, mangoes, papayas, and avocados, will not juice well. They can be used in smoothies and cold soups by first juicing other produce, then pouring the juice into a blender and adding the avocado, for example, to make a raw soup.

- *Drink your juice as soon as you can after it's made.* If you can't drink the juice right away, store it in an insulated container such as a stainless steel water bottle, thermos, or another airtight, opaque container in the refrigerator for up to twenty-four hours. Light, heat, and air will destroy nutrients quickly. Be aware that the longer juice sits before you drink it, the more nutrients are lost. If juice turns brown, it has oxidized and lost a large amount of its nutritional value. After twenty-four hours it may become spoiled. I must add, however, that when I was very sick with chronic fatigue syndrome, I only had enough energy to juice midday. I would store some of the juice for up to twenty-four hours. I got well doing that, so I know the juice had plenty of nutrients even in the stored amount. Melon and cabbage juices do not store well; drink them soon after they've been juiced.

Chapter 4

The Weekend Weight-Loss Diet

WELCOME TO THE Weekend Weight-Loss Diet—the jump-start program for weight loss on a healthy mission. You're off to a great start! And like so many others who've used this plan to embark on a healthy lifestyle, you too will be amazed at how you feel.

If you think you will have nothing interesting left to eat on this diet, you will be happily surprised. The two-day plan includes drinking delicious veggie juice made from the low-glycemic, great-tasting recipes in chapter 7. And because I'm so sure you'll love the way you look and feel after the first two days, as a bonus, I've also included recipes and a menu plan for delicious foods, juices, and smoothies that give you the option to extend this into a fourteen-day plan. Why? Because I want you to think of this weekend as the launch of a lifetime of healthful eating. It's your "lighthouse" on the troubled sea of bad food choices luring you away from your best and highest goals. If you stray, it's the way to pilot home and return to your life-giving choices.

Since you're about to embark on a liquid diet for the next two days, I'd like to share a few pointers about the different types of liquids I do and do not recommend. First, avoid processed fruit juices; they become more acid producing when processed and especially when sweetened. Freshly made raw, vegetable juices are alkaline producing, and achieving a healthy alkaline-acid balance through your diet and lifestyle is critically important to weight loss and health.

Juice Every Day

Even when you aren't on a juicing diet, my recommendation is that you drink two glasses of veggie juice each day. It's best to drink one glass of veggie juice in the morning and one in the afternoon or before dinner. The morning juice helps energize your body and gives you super nutrients to last all morning; the afternoon juice is a pick-me-up for the afternoon slump many people experience.

You can also add another glass of veggie juice in the evening (as a before-dinner cocktail). This helps curb your appetite and gives you energy to make a healthy dinner.

If you plan to do the Weekend Weight-Loss Diet during a busy weekend or even during the work week, remember that you can make your juice the night before and take juice to work or weekend activities in a stainless steel water bottle or thermos. You can store juice in a covered container in the refrigerator up to twenty-four hours. Some people prefer to make enough for the entire day at once and store in a gallon-size container and drink that throughout the day. That will give you plenty of juice so you won't be hungry.

Green tea is another great addition to your healthy lifestyle while you're on the Weekend Weight-Loss Diet. Rich in antioxidants and the phytonutrients catechins and other polyphenols that protect against inflammation, cancer, and other ailments, green tea is also thermogenic. For these reasons it's a great idea to make green tea part of your daily meal plan. Strive for at least one cup of organic green tea per day. A cup of green tea has about one-third of the caffeine found in a cup of coffee. Avoid green tea if you are sensitive to caffeine, have low adrenal function, or are hypoglycemic.

White tea has less caffeine than green tea and may be better tolerated. Herbal teas are also a great choice and are fine for those with low adrenal function and who are hypoglycemic. When choosing green, white, and herbal tea, look for organically grown. And unbleached tea bags are a better choice over bleached.

Be sure to drink plenty of water. It's recommended that you drink at least eight 8-ounce glasses of purified water per day for weight loss and to maintain good health. A good water purifier is a great investment. Be aware of plastic toxins that are leached into the water from the plastic bottles. Take water with you in stainless steel water bottles.

To make the cranberry water you'll see listed in the menu plans, start with unsweetened cranberry juice—just juice, nothing added. Add 1–2 tablespoons of cranberry juice or cranberry concentrate to an 8-ounce glass of purified water. Adjust cranberry juice to taste. You may add a few drops of stevia as desired.

Sparkling mineral water may be substituted for water at any time. You may add a squeeze of lemon or lime for added flavor, or unsweetened cranberry juice. For sparkling water, choose mineral water that is naturally carbonated, such as S. Pellegrino and Apollinaris, over commercially gassed varieties. If you suffer from IBS, Crohn's disease, celiac, or diverticulitis, it is advisable to completely eliminate carbonated drinks along with all gluten from your diet in order to allow the GI lining of your intestinal tract to heal.

Completely avoid soft drinks; they are like drinking liquid candy with chemicals so caustic they can rust nails. They're loaded with sugar or artificial sweeteners that are even worse. Studies have connected them with weight gain and numerous health problems. They're also very acidic. Also, watch out for sweetened teas, energy drinks, sports drinks, and vitamin-infused water. And always avoid diet sodas due to their detrimental health effects and the fact that they actually cause people to gain weight.

THE ONE-DAY JUMP-START JUICE CLEANSE

To accelerate weight loss or get a jump start on your health, try my One-Day Jump-Start Juice Cleanse or my Weekend Weight-Loss Diet. I'll outline both programs for you here.

For the One-Day Jump-Start Juice Cleanse you can pick a day you are off from work to make it more convenient for you, or you can juice ahead and take your juice to work. Some people like to have juice for dinner the night before and breakfast and lunch the next day, with a meal that evening. Some people repeat a juice cleanse every week on the same day to keep their bodies cleansed of toxins and pumped full of nutrition. Choose what works for you.

This daylong liquid diet helps you detox your body and flush out fat. During this day you will only drink vegetable juice, vegetable broth, water, sparkling mineral water, and herbal, green, or white tea. Here's a sample plan to take you through the day.

Day 1

Breakfast

- Green, white, or herbal tea with lemon juice or hot water with lemon and a dash of cayenne pepper (this helps the liver get moving)
- Juice of choice

Midmorning

- 9:30 a.m.: 8 ounces of water or cranberry water
- 10:30 a.m.: Juice of choice
- 11:30 a.m.: Green, white, or herbal tea or 8 ounces of water or sparkling mineral water

Lunch

- Juice of choice

Midafternoon

- 1:30 p.m.: 8 ounces of water or cranberry water
- 2:30 p.m.: 8 ounces of water or cranberry water
- 3:00 p.m.: Juice of choice
- 4:00 p.m.: 8 ounces of water or cranberry water
- 5:00 p.m.: 8 ounces of water or cranberry water

Dinner

- Juice of choice (you may also add a cup of warm vegetable broth)
- Cup of herbal tea

The Weekend Weight-Loss Diet

If you're doing the weekend version, start Friday evening with juice or a smoothie for dinner, and follow the meal plan for Saturday and breakfast and lunch on Sunday. Then choose a raw food recipe for your Sunday dinner.

Note: If you find that you are too spacey or your blood sugar drops too low while on the Weekend Weight-Loss Diet, add a bowl of quick-energy soup such as Cherie's Yummy Energy Soup or a green smoothie for one meal. Here's a meal plan to follow for the entire weekend or any two days you choose. (All of the recipes suggested below are found in chapter 7 of this book.)

Friday

Dinner

- Juice or smoothie of choice, such as Cran-Apple Cocktail
- Cup of herbal tea

Saturday

Breakfast

- Green, white, or herbal tea with lemon juice or hot water with lemon and a dash of cayenne pepper (this helps the liver get moving)
- Juice of choice, such as Green Berry Blast or Energize-Your-Day Cocktail

Midmorning

- 9:30 a.m.: 8 ounces of water or cranberry water
- 10:30 a.m.: Juice of choice, such as Triple C
- 11:30 a.m.: Green, white, or herbal tea or 8 ounces of water or sparkling mineral water

Lunch

- Juice of choice, such as You Are Loved Cocktail or Green Lemonade

Midafternoon

- 1:30 p.m.: 8 ounces of water, lemon water, or cranberry water
- 2:30 p.m.: 8 ounces of water, lemon water, or cranberry water
- 3:00 p.m.: Vegetable juice of choice, such as Arugula Cocktail
- 4:00 p.m.: 8 ounces of water, lemon water, or cranberry water
- 5:00 p.m.: 8 ounces of water, lemon water, or cranberry water

Dinner

- Juice of choice, such as Weight-Loss Buddy (you may also add a cup of warm vegetable broth)
- Cup of herbal tea

Sunday

Breakfast

- Green, white, or herbal tea with lemon juice or hot water with lemon and a dash of cayenne pepper (this helps the liver get moving)
- Juice of choice, such as Pink Morning

Midmorning

- 9:30 a.m.: 8 ounces of water or cranberry water
- 10:30 a.m.: Juice of choice, such as Tomato Florentine
- 11:30 a.m.: Green, white, or herbal tea or 8 ounces of water or sparkling mineral water

Lunch

- Juice of choice, such as Tomato and Spice

Midafternoon

- 1:30 p.m.: 8 ounces of water, lemon water, or cranberry water
- 2:30 p.m.: 8 ounces of water, lemon water, or cranberry water
- 3:00 p.m.: Vegetable juice of choice, such as Beet, Carrot, Coconut Blast
- 4:00 p.m.: 8 ounces of water, lemon water, or cranberry water

- 5:00 p.m.: 8 ounces of water, lemon water, or cranberry water

Dinner

- Soup, salad, or main course raw food entrée of choice
- Cup of herbal tea

BONUS! Extend Your Weight-Loss Program to Two Full Weeks

If Sunday evening rolls around and your Weekend Weight-Loss Diet has you looking and feeling great, you will likely want to keep that momentum going! I encourage you to get a copy of my book *The Juice Lady's Living Foods Revolution*, which will set you on the path to healthy eating for life by incorporating more juices, smoothies, and raw foods into your diet. But for now, if you want to extend your juice-based diet beyond the weekend, while slowly adding solid foods back into your diet, follow this bonus meal plan. (All of the recipes suggested below are found in chapter 7 of this book.)

Monday

Breakfast

- Juice of choice, such as Happy Mood Morning
- Apple Muesli
- Green, white, or herbal tea (and a squeeze of lemon is nice)

Midmorning snack

- Juice of choice, herbal tea, or cranberry water
- Half dozen sun-dried or naturally processed green or black organic olives

Lunch

- Mock "Salmon" Pate with Raw Almond Mayo
- 2–3 Flax Crackers

Midafternoon snack

- Juice of choice or cranberry water
- Veggie sticks with 1 tablespoon raw almond butter

Dinner

- Juice of choice, such as The Ginger Hopper With a Twist
- Almond Roulade
- Marinated Collard Greens

Tuesday

Breakfast

- Juice of choice, such as Cranberry-Pear Fat Buster
- Green, white, or herbal tea (and a squeeze of lemon is nice)

Midmorning snack

- Juice of choice, herbal tea, or cranberry water
- 12 raw almonds

Lunch

- Red Bell Pepper Soup
- Sliced tomatoes with extra-virgin olive oil and balsamic vinegar
- 2–3 Veggie Nut Crackers

Midafternoon snack

- Juice of choice, herbal tea, or cranberry water

- Piece of low-sugar fruit such as a green apple

Dinner

- Juice of choice, such as Goin' Green
- Sliced cucumbers with balsamic vinegar
- Raw Zucchini Noodles With Marinara Sauce

Wednesday

Breakfast

- Juice of choice, such as The Morning Energizer
- Lemon Muesli with oat, almond, or rice milk
- Green, white, or herbal tea (and a squeeze of lemon is nice)

Midmorning snack

- Juice of choice, herbal tea, or cranberry water
- 2 tablespoons raw sunflower seeds

Lunch

- Winter Salad
- 1–2 Nan's Carrot Curry Flax Krax

Midafternoon snack

- Juice of choice, herbal tea, or cranberry water
- 2 tablespoons raw sunflower seeds

Dinner

- Juice of choice, such as Peppy Parsley
- Mexican Almond Dip
- Awesome Corn Crackers

- Chef Avi Dalene's Green Tortillas with Nan's Sunflower Pate and Mango Salsa or tomato salsa

Thursday

Breakfast

- Juice of choice, such as Happy Mood Morning
- Sprouted Buckwheat Groats with milk of choice and ground nuts or raw seeds
- Green, white, or herbal tea (and a squeeze of lemon is nice)

Midmorning snack

- Juice of choice, herbal tea, or cranberry water
- Granny Smith or Pippin apple or veggie sticks

Lunch

- Sprouted Quinoa Salad
- 2–3 Veggie Nut Crackers

Midafternoon snack

- Juice of choice, herbal tea, or cranberry water
- 6 raw almonds

Dinner

- Juice of choice, such as Green Recharger
- Gourmet Pesto Pizza
- Sliced tomatoes with extra-virgin olive oil and balsamic vinegar

Friday

Breakfast

- Smoothie of choice, such as Kale-Pear Smoothie
- Green, white, or herbal tea (and a squeeze of lemon is nice)

Midmorning snack

- Juice of choice, herbal tea, or cranberry water
- Zucchini Hummus with 2 Awesome Corn Crackers

Lunch

- Almond Falafel with Sunflower Dill Sauce
- Icy Spicy Gazpacho

Midafternoon snack

- Juice of choice, herbal tea, or cranberry water
- 1 Granny Smith or Pippin apple

Dinner

- Juice of choice, such as South of the Border Cocktail
- Sunny Delight Enchiladas With Corn Tortillas with Mango Salsa
- Green salad with dressing of choice

Saturday

Breakfast

- Smoothie of choice, such as Berry Blast Smoothie
- and/or
- Green Coconut Delight with raw sunflower seeds

- Green, white, or herbal tea (and a squeeze of lemon is nice)

Midmorning snack

- Juice of choice, herbal tea, or cranberry water
- Boiled egg or 2 tablespoons of raw seeds or nuts

Lunch

- Salad (with option of chicken strips or broiled salmon)
- 1–2 Awesome Corn Crackers

Midafternoon snack

- Juice of choice, herbal tea, or cranberry water
- Veggie sticks

Dinner

- Juice of choice, such as Springtime Tonic
- Salad with Sesame Dressing
- Carrot Sauce With Asparagus and Fresh Peas Over Rice

Sunday

Breakfast

- Juice of choice, such as Pink Morning
- Buckwheat Granola or old-fashioned oatmeal with almond, oat, or rice milk
- Green, white, or herbal tea (and a squeeze of lemon is nice)

Midmorning snack

- Juice of choice, herbal tea, or cranberry water
- Veggie sticks

Lunch

- Borscht in the Raw or Vegetable Medley
- Dr. Nina's Russian Cabbage Slaw

Midafternoon snack

- Juice of choice, herbal tea, or cranberry water
- Spicy Kale Chips

Dinner

- Juice of choice, such as Twisted Ginger
- Stir-fry with brown and wild rice
- Green salad with Ginger-Lime Dressing

Monday

Breakfast

- Juice of choice, such as Refreshing Mint Cocktail
- Apple Muesli
- Green, white, or herbal tea (and a squeeze of lemon is nice)

Midmorning snack

- Juice of choice, herbal tea, or cranberry water
- Half dozen sun-dried or naturally processed green or black organic olives

Lunch

- Main course salad of choice with cup of chili or soup of choice
- 2–3 Flax Crackers

Midafternoon snack

- Juice of choice, herbal tea, or cranberry water
- Veggie sticks with 1 tablespoon raw almond butter

Dinner

- Juice of choice, such as Waldorf Twist
- Squash and Arugula Enchiladas
- Marinated Collard Greens

Tuesday

Breakfast

- Juice or smoothie of choice, such as Nutty Delight
- Green, white, or herbal tea (and a squeeze of lemon is nice)

Midmorning snack

- Juice of choice or herbal tea
- 12 raw almonds

Lunch

- Creamy Red Pepper Soup or salad of choice
- Sliced tomatoes with extra-virgin olive oil and balsamic vinegar
- 2–3 Nan's Zesty Green Berry Krax

Midafternoon snack

- Juice of choice, herbal tea, or cranberry water
- Piece of low-sugar fruit such as a green apple

Dinner

- Juice of choice, such as Greens of Life
- Sliced cucumbers with balsamic vinegar
- Nicole's Stuffed Acorn Squash

Wednesday

Breakfast

- Juice of choice, such as Liver-Cleansing Cocktail
- Green, white, or herbal tea (and a squeeze of lemon is nice)

Midmorning snack

- Juice of choice or herbal tea
- 2 tablespoons raw sunflower seeds

Lunch

- Apple Fennel Salad With Lemon Zest
- 2–3 Nan's Zesty Green Berry Krax

Midafternoon snack

- Juice of choice, herbal tea, or cranberry water
- 2 tablespoons raw sunflower seeds

Dinner

- Juice of choice, such as Super Green Sprout Drink
- Garlic Dijon Halibut
- Steamed vegetable such as broccoli or brussels sprouts
- Green salad with dressing of choice

Thursday

Breakfast

- Juice of choice, such as Mood Mender
- Guilt-Free "Bacon"
- Sliced tomatoes or sliced avocado
- Green, white, or herbal tea (and a squeeze of lemon is nice)

Midmorning snack

- Juice of choice (optional)
- Celery sticks with 1 teaspoon almond butter

Lunch

- Cherie's Yummy Energy Soup
- Sliced tomatoes with extra-virgin olive oil and balsamic vinegar
- 2–3 Nan's Zesty Green Berry Krax

Midafternoon snack

- Juice of choice (optional)
- Veggie sticks

Dinner

- Juice of choice, such as Veggie Time Cocktail
- Stuffed Bell Peppers
- Sliced tomatoes with extra-virgin olive oil and balsamic vinegar

Friday

Breakfast

- Smoothie of choice, such as Healthy Green Smoothie

- Fresh or frozen berries: blueberries, blackberries, or strawberries
- Green, white, or herbal tea (and a squeeze of lemon is nice)

Midmorning snack

- Juice of choice, herbal tea, or cranberry water
- Dehydrated tomato slices

Lunch

- Eggless Salad Roll-ups
- 2–3 Nan's Zesty Green Berry Krax

Midafternoon snack

- Juice of choice, herbal tea, or cranberry water
- 1 Granny Smith or Pippin apple

Dinner

- Juice of choice, such as Green Delight
- Walnut Zucchini Greens
- Cherie's Nut Burgers

GOING VEGAN?

When you've reached your weight-loss goals, you may be wondering if a vegetarian or vegan lifestyle is right for you. I advocate incorporating as many raw plant foods into your life as possible, but I do understand that we're all different. Some find optimum health in a vegan lifestyle; some do not. Some need muscle meats in their diet, while others thrive without any. Regardless of which side you end up on, we can all agree that no one needs a lot of meat, but we all need a lot of vegetables. And the more veggies we consume raw, the more vibrantly healthy we become. If you want to glow with health, this is your path.

And everyone can do short-term "raw vegan weeks" for cleansing and detoxifying your system. Also, a one- or two-day vegetable juice fast occasionally is very helpful for cleansing the body, which leads me to my final thought for this chapter.

WHEN TO REPEAT THE ONE- OR TWO-DAY DIET

Eventually, you'll be celebrating the achievement of your weight-loss goals. When that day comes, you can slowly add more healthy carbohydrates, including whole grains, potatoes, squash, and fruit to your diet. Typically in this phase you will lose about a pound per week. If you eat too many of these higher carb foods or you splurge for holidays, vacations, or special occasions and gain weight, you can quickly lose those extra pounds by cleansing your body with the One-Day Jump-Start Juice Cleanse or the Weekend Weight-Loss Diet. If you trip up and binge during a stressful time, you can schedule a vegetable juice cleanse day and flush out the toxins. This is the design that can help you maintain your ideal weight for the rest of your life.

BEYOND THE WEEKEND: TIPS FOR WEIGHT-LOSS SUCCESS

Cut your calories. Most people lose weight when they embark on a juicing program because they lose cravings for junk food and high-carb foods. But make sure that you shave off at least one hundred calories from your daily caloric intake. All long-term weight studies ever done where people kept the weight off for more than two years showed this simple strategy. And it's very easy to do. Further, one hundred calories is such a small amount your body won't be able to tell that you're on a diet. This way your metabolism doesn't slow down, and you naturally lose weight. But don't worry if you're shaving off more than one hundred calories a day on a living foods diet, which will probably happen. Your metabolism should not slow down because this style of eating is replete with living nutrients such as vitamins, enzymes, and biophotons that rev up your metabolism.

Eat breakfast. If you think skipping breakfast will cut a bunch of calories from your diet and speed your weight loss, you're mistaken. People who skip breakfast usually eat more for lunch because they're so hungry, and they usually snack more throughout the day. Start your day with a power breakfast—first a glass of raw veggie juice and/or a green smoothie, a nut smoothie, or another living foods dish. Many people say they just aren't hungry after drinking an energizing glass of veggie juice or green smoothie. That may be all you want, but if you're still hungry, follow with some protein such as raw nuts or seeds, raw veggie dip and fresh vegetables, a vegetable omelet, or bowl of old-fashioned steel cut oatmeal. In a study of people who dropped at least thirty pounds, 78 percent said they ate breakfast.[1] Make sure you eat something within an hour of rising, which will boost your metabolism by 10 percent.

Eat healthy snacks. Each day, if you work outside the home, pack healthy snacks in small containers or plastic bags to take with you and keep in your purse, briefcase, or an insulated tote. If you always have healthy diet-friendly snacks such as fresh veggies, low-sugar fruit, raw nuts, or seeds on hand, you'll be less tempted to raid the vending machine or grab a few pieces of candy from a coworker's dish. And you won't go home ravenously hungry and eat half a bag of chips or cookies before dinner.

Drink purified water. The next time you feel hungry, drink a glass of purified water, and you may not need to eat. Since the hormones in our intestinal tract tell us we're hungry and are very similar to the hormones that let us know we're thirsty, it's often hard to distinguish hunger from thirst. Therefore, we reach for food when we should be reaching for water. Your hunger pangs could be your body's cry for H_2O. Water is essential for burning calories. People who drink eight or more glasses of water a day burn more calories than those who drink less.[2] If you don't like the taste of plain water, add fresh lemon juice. I like lemon and ginger juice added to the water. (My husband and I each drink about a quart of that combination a day.) You may also want to invest in a good water purifier. It's amazing how that improves the taste and purity of the water, which equates to better health.

Go low glycemic. Low-glycemic diet plans, also known as low-carb, are popular for a reason—they get results. High-glycemic foods raise blood sugar levels, cause the body to secrete excess insulin, and lead to the storage of fat. Originally developed as a tool to help diabetics manage blood sugar, the low-glycemic diet has become popular in the weight-loss market largely because it works so well. The *Journal of the American Medical Association* reported that patients who lost weight with a low-glycemic diet kept the weight off longer than patients who lost the same amount of weight with a standard low-fat diet.[3] Low-fat dieting is not good for your body. We need adequate amounts of essential fats such as omega-3s. Make quality fats about 30 percent of your diet, which will also contribute to satiety—that feeling of satisfaction and that you've had enough to eat.

Keep a positive attitude. Never tell yourself that you can't do something such as lose weight. Remove all negative thoughts from your mind; speak and think only positive words to yourself and others. If you have a five-pound reduction goal by the end of two weeks, see those five pounds gone. Think about this in terms of what you want to weigh by the end of two weeks. How great will you feel when you are five pounds lighter? Guard against self-defeat. Don't let it get you before you even get started.

Here are some additional tips after the weekend is over to propel your weight-loss success into high gear.

- Drink a minimum of two 10- to 12-ounce glasses of vegetable juice every day.

- For the best success, strive to eat between 75 and 80 percent of your foods raw. (Foods that have been dehydrated between 105 and 115 degrees are considered raw because the enzymes and vitamins have not been destroyed with heat.)

- For at least the first three weeks, omit all starchy vegetables such as potatoes, yams, winter squash, corn, and peas. Also, omit all grains. You can have wild rice; it's actually a cereal grass and is lower in carbohydrates.

- Limit nuts for snacks to no more than a dozen per day and seeds to no more than 1 or 2 tablespoons; nut butters to about 1 teaspoon. Nuts contain carbohydrates.

- Make one day a week a juice feast day. On this day, consume only vegetable juices and raw soups along with the water quota and green, white, or herbal tea.

- Drink eight to ten glasses of purified water every day. If you add a little cranberry juice or cranberry concentrate to the water, it will help to flush fat and will also act as a diuretic. Buy pure, unsweetened cranberry juice or cranberry juice concentrate. This also helps to curb your appetite.

- Have a small snack or glass of vegetable juice in the midmorning and midafternoon. This will help to keep your blood sugar stable so that you won't be tempted to overeat at lunch or eat snack foods before dinner or overeat at your evening meal.

- The lighter the evening meal, the faster you will lose weight, because we don't typically burn as many calories in the evening as we do during the day.

- Develop an exercise plan that includes a varied workout three to four times a week.

Chapter 5

In the Produce Aisle
(Shopping Guide)

THIS CHAPTER IS your shopping guide—your manual of sorts—to lead you through the endless options of unhealthy foodstuffs that line the shelves and freezers of our supermarkets. All animal products are not the same; neither are vegetables and fruit, nor anything else for that matter.

The mission of *The Juice Lady's Weekend Weight-Loss Diet* is to help you get a jump start on eating healthier, losing weight if you need to, detoxifying your body, and preventing disease by choosing living foods that are also clean, fresh, whole foods. These are the foods that give your body life.

Because the majority of the food in typical grocery stores does not give the body life, smart shopping is the key to healthy eating. And planning ahead is the best way to avoid making poor food choices when there's nothing around to eat and you feel half starved. If you make meal plans and shop ahead of time, you'll have food on hand and an idea for when and how you'll make the food. This will give you a much better chance of succeeding after you've jump-started your weight loss.

If something unexpected comes your way, have a backup plan for something nutritious you can thaw out, dehydrated foods already made, or something you can quickly put together. To this end the information in this chapter will help you make the wisest choices.

Choose Real, Whole Food

More and more we hear the term *real foods* or *whole foods*, which are meant to counter substances that are man-made—whipped up in factories and spun out in forms that are anything but real or whole. These foods have become the basis of the American diet, but they should not be called food and should not be part of anyone's diet. They are processed and depleted of natural nutrients and filled with chemicals to promote longer shelf life, ease of transportation, and longer storage. Despite a variety of flavors, textures, and shapes, most of these products are manufactured from the same mono-cultured crops—wheat, corn, soy, and potatoes. They are depleted in nutrients due to growth in high-density environments and depleted soils, while also being saturated with petroleum-based fertilizers. These are among the biggest genetically modified crops (GMO) in America. Due to this stressful growth situation, they are susceptible to pests. Commercial agriculture deals with their susceptibility by spraying them with high amounts of insecticides or by producing GMO frankenplants that have pesticides built in such as Monsanto's Roundup Ready alfalfa. This poses alarming threats to our ecosystem, our long-term food supply, and our health.

Plant nutrient values are further diminished in the course of processing and storage, so the processed foods are fortified with synthetic vitamins and minerals. And flavorings are added to improve the taste because they have very little flavor left. These foods are often addictive and carcinogenic, while being void of nutrients necessary for cellular function. And they deliver empty calories that get stored as fat because the body can't use them for most of its functions.

These products become the basis of disease, obesity, reduced immunity, and reduced fertility, making Americans *the most* overfed and undernourished nation in the world.

Real foods are the foods that are the least processed. They are closest to their natural form and, therefore, retain the most nutrient value and deliver the highest health benefits. They are picked after they've ripened, and they are rich in flavor. They retain natural diversity of taste. They have full nutrient and antioxidant content. And if they are organically grown, seasonal, and local foods, they are the healthiest choices possible.

FRUIT, VEGETABLES, AND LEGUMES

In order to choose the very best fruit, vegetables, and legumes, opt for the freshest produce you can find that has been grown organically to avoid toxic pesticides and to get increased nutrition. Buy from local growers whenever possible, because that produce is fresher than anything trucked in from other locations. Many local growers will deliver a box of produce to your door each week. Just check out websites for organic growers in your area. And if you select the produce in season, that's about the freshest food you'll be able to find. And the fresher the produce, the more vitamins and biophotons you'll get.

Vegetables and fruit selected off the shelf at a grocery store usually emit fewer biophotons because of loss during transportation and storage. Chemical, gas, or heat treatment, which is used to ripen or preserve fruits and vegetables, further reduces the amount of biophotons and nutrients available. Irradiation, which is radiation treatment with gamma rays in order to increase the shelf life of food, leads to total destruction of biophotons and many nutrients. (I will discuss irradiation further a little later in this chapter.)

We might be buying attractive fruits and veggies at the market, but their biophoton, enzyme, and vitamin content may be close to zero. For example, avocados may be heat treated in order to speed up ripening, but if the heat is above 110 degrees, it kills enzymes, vitamins, and biophotons—the life force of the cells. Most almonds are required to be pasteurized. But even *raw* almonds may actually have undergone pasteurization, thereby eliminating their biophoton content and reducing their nutrients. The freshest produce can be found at farmers markets, local farms, and your own backyard, along with foraging wild greens. It may be that some day the healthiest food we can find will be unsprayed dandelions in our own backyard.

The quality of protein in vegetables is related to the amount of nitrogen in the soil. Conventional chemical fertilizers add extra nitrogen, which increases the amount of protein but creates a reduction in its quality. Organically managed soils release nitrogen in smaller amounts over a longer time than conventional fertilizers. As a result, the quality of protein from organic crops is better in terms of human nutrition. Indeed, studies show that across the board, organically grown produce is higher in nutrients.[1] (I'll discuss more information on the compelling reasons to purchase organic produce later in this chapter.)

Choose heirloom and wild plants as often as possible. The more of these plants that we eat, the more high-quality nutrition we get. Also, when commercial plants are hybridized, they lose more and more of their inherent biological information contained in the DNA. This is what also makes them more susceptible to the onslaught of diseases, insects, and parasites. Then farmers are told they need to spray their crops with highly toxic chemicals to kill the pests. It's a destructive cycle that affects our health in the end. The more nutrient-rich foods you eat, the more satisfied you'll be and the more cravings will diminish. That will have a positive impact on your health and weight management. Also, this will have positive benefits for farmworkers, the animals, and our earth.

Wild foods. Wild foods such as dandelion greens, nettles, wood sorrel, wild salad greens, and shepherd's purse offer us nutrients found nowhere else. Consider also that if people have adapted to eating wild plants for several hundred thousand years, then problems may arise when we try to eat hybridized and genetically engineered fruits and veggies. Our physiology is just not programmed to handle this.

Vegetables. I encourage you to eat lots of brightly colored vegetables since they are packed with satisfying nutrients. Eat plenty of energy soups, salads, sprouts, vegetable sticks, and steamed vegetables, along with drinking veggie juices and green smoothies and eating raw food dishes. Avoid baked vegetables as much as possible since the sugar content is highest when they're baked. Limit high-starch vegetables such as potatoes, yams, and acorn squash to no more than three times per week when you're trying to lose weight. If you're dining out or it's a special occasion, and you just can't resist a potato, the best choice is red potatoes (less carbs). If you do succumb to a baked potato, which is very high in carbs, eat it with a little fat such as butter. This will help to slow down the rate at which sugar enters your bloodstream.

Fruit. Four of the best fruits you can choose are lemons, limes (both very alkaline), avocado, and tomato. Avocados are an excellent source of essential fatty acids and glutathione (a powerful antioxidant), along with some protein. They contain more potassium than bananas, making them an excellent choice for heart disorders. Tomatoes are a rich source of vitamin C, beta-carotene, potassium, molybdenum, and one of the best sources of lycopene. The antioxidant function of lycopene includes its ability to help protect cells and other structures in the body from oxygen damage. It has been linked in human research to the protection of DNA (our genetic material) inside of white blood cells. Lycopene also plays a role in the prevention of heart disease. To get the most lycopene, choose organic tomatoes.

To avoid getting too much sugar, choose the lowest glycemic fruit such as lemons, limes, berries, cantaloupe, cherries, grapefruit, and apples (especially green). Only purchase organic for most of these fruits because they're heavily sprayed. Be aware of eating too much fruit except for lemons and limes. Cranberries are another excellent low-sugar fruit. Buy them in the fall and freeze some for when they're out of season. They contain iodine, which is good for the thyroid. If you buy store-bought cranberry juice, look for unsweetened cranberry concentrate or pure cranberry juice. (Of the bottled juices, cranberry contains the least amount of fungus.) Add lemon, lime, or cranberry juice to flavor water and juices.

Legumes. Legumes (beans, lentils, dried peas) are packed with nutrition, including protein, calcium, vitamins, and minerals. And they are very cheap. When cooked right, they are delicious. They can also be sprouted. Legumes offer a lot of health benefits. They help prevent food cravings, metabolic syndrome, type 2 diabetes, and obesity. That's because the outer casing of legumes, which is high fiber, slows down the rate at which sugar enters your bloodstream. Legumes also protect the body against cancer and heart disease. Further, they provide lots of protein for energy

Why Choose Organic Produce?

The Environmental Protection Agency (EPA) considers 60 percent of herbicides, 90 percent of fungicides, and 30 percent of insecticides to be carcinogenic, and most are damaging to the nervous system as well.[2] Pesticide residues pose long-term health risks, such as cancer, Alzheimer's, Parkinson's, male infertility, miscarriages, and birth defects, along with immediate health risks to farmers and farmworkers from acute intoxication such as vomiting, diarrhea, blurred vision, tremors, and convulsions.[3]

Many pesticides that are known or suspected to cause brain and nervous system damage, cancer, disruption of the endocrine and immune systems, and a host of other toxic effects are in our food supply. Though the cancer-causing pesticide Alar was banned twenty years ago, we are still no better protected.

There is a far greater incidence of cancer, particularly lymphoma, leukemia, and cancer of the brain, skin, stomach, and prostate among farmers, their families, and farmworkers when compared with cancer rates among the general public.[4] This data alone should be alarming enough to ban all pesticides in America. But there are huge profits at stake for big corporations that lobby hard in Washington, pay for studies to show that their pesticides aren't that harmful, and "educate" farmers on the merits of pesticides, making them believe that we would not have enough food to feed people if it weren't for pesticides.

This is far from true. Our local co-op (PCC) published an excellent article in their *Sound Consumer* paper in September 2010 titled "Organic Can Feed the World." Author Maria Rodale states, "Biotech and chemical companies have spent billions of dollars trying to make us think that synthetic fertilizers, pesticides, and genetically modified organisms (GMO) are necessary to feed a growing population. But science indicates otherwise. There's clear and conclusive scientific data showing organic agriculture is key not only to solving global hunger but also to...promoting public health, revitalizing farming communities, and restoring the environment."[5]

Research by the Rodale Institute called the Farm System Trial (FST), which began in 1981, shows that once soil is restored organically from depletion due to years of mismanagement, organic crops yield comparable to yields using chemicals. The study also found that organic farm yields are higher during times of drought and floods due to stronger root systems and better moisture retention. The FST data also showed that organic production requires 30 percent less energy than chemical production for growing corn and soybeans. They also found that organic production stores a great deal of carbon and concluded that if we returned globally to organic farming, we could reduce our CO_2 pollution significantly. These findings are supported by the $12 million study by the International Assessment of Agricultural Knowledge, Science, and Technology for Development.[6]

When you purchase produce from certified organic farmers or from local farmers who sell unsprayed produce but are working without certification, you won't get synthetic fertilizers, sewage sludge, genetically modified organisms, or ionizing radiation. Buying your vegetables from a local source is also the best way to insure freshness. Keep in mind that the fresher the vegetables and fruit, the more biophotons you'll be receiving. Many local farmers will deliver a box of organic produce each week for a very reasonable price. We have fresh organic veggies delivered to our door, and it's always a nice surprise to see what we'll get that week. The vegetables we get differ from week to week. If you sign up for such a program, there may be items in the box you've never eaten before, which is great! You'll get to try something new. And that's the best way to get maximum nutrition—by varying your foods and not eating the same things all the time.

Is Organic Food More Nutritious?

I'm often asked if organic produce is more nutritious than conventionally grown fruits and vegetables. Studies have shown that it is. According to results from a $25 million study into organic food, the largest of its kind to date, organic produce completely surpasses conventional produce in nutritional content. A four-year, European Union–funded study in 2007 found that organic fruits and vegetables contain up to 40 percent more antioxidants. They have higher levels of beneficial minerals such as iron and zinc. Milk from organic herds contained up to 90 percent more antioxidants. The researchers obtained their results after growing fruits and vegetables and raising cattle on adjacent organic and nonorganic sites attached to Newcastle University. According to Professor Carlo Leifert, coordinator of the project, eating organic foods can even help to increase the nutrient intake of people who don't eat the recommended number of servings of fruits and vegetables a day.[7]

Additionally, a 2001 study completed as part of a doctoral dissertation at Johns Hopkins University looked at forty-one different studies involving field trials, greenhouse pot experiments, market basket surveys, and surveys of farmers. The most studied nutrients across those surveys included calcium, copper, iron, magnesium, manganese, phosphorus, potassium, sodium, zinc, beta-carotene, and vitamin C. Many studies also looked at nitrates. According to the study, there was significantly more vitamin C (27 percent), iron (21 percent), magnesium (29 percent), and phosphorus (13 percent) in the organic produce than in the conventionally grown vegetables. There were also 15 percent fewer nitrates in the organic vegetables. The vegetables that had the largest increases in nutrients between organic and conventional production were lettuce, spinach, carrots, potatoes, and cabbage.[8] Couple that with fewer chemical residues, and you can see that buying organically grown food is well worth the effort and the additional cost. Plus, you're investing in sustainability of farming and the health of the entire human community as well as our earth.

Studies Reveal Pesticides and Other Toxins Make Us Fat

Researchers showed that the common herbicide atrazine causes sex changes in fish, and it also makes rats fat regardless of their feeding behavior. "It's possible that the sorts of genes that play a role in reading signals on the way from the brain to the periphery to regulate fat are being acted upon by pesticides and...things that are in the environment," said Kaveh Ashrafi, MD, PhD.

Dr. Ashrafi mentioned another study in which mice were exposed for five days to diethylstilbestrol (DES)—used in feed for factory-farm livestock and poultry—while in utero. The mice had normal birth weights and normal growth rates, but they ended up much fatter over time even though they had the same eating and activity habits as mice that were not exposed to DES.

Could drug residues in commercial meat be contributing to weight gain for people who eat commercial animal products frequently? Dr. Ashrafi said, "Maybe environmental toxins are essentially drugs that we are taking without knowing it, and they're acting in this process to promote fat regulation."[9]

BUYING ORGANIC: HOW TO CHOOSE THE BEST

When choosing organically grown foods, look for labels that are marked *certified organic*. This means the produce has been cultivated according to strict uniform standards that are verified by independent state or private organizations. Certification includes inspection of farms and processing facilities, detailed record keeping, and pesticide testing of soil and water to ensure that growers and handlers are meeting government standards. But there are a couple of categories where there's evidence that standards may be getting lax with dairy products and the labeling of some packaged foods.

Support your local farms and farmers who sell their produce at farmers markets, local markets, and home deliveries. Many of the smaller farms can't promote their wares as "organic," but if you talk with them, you'll learn that they don't use pesticides or chemical fertilizers; they just can't afford to get certified.

You may occasionally see a label that says *transitional organic*. This means that the produce was grown on a farm that recently converted or is in the process of converting from chemical sprays and fertilizer to organic farming. It's always a good idea to support these farmers.

If you are not able to afford to purchase everything organic, avoid the worst offenders. According to the Environmental

Working Group, commercially farmed fruits and vegetables vary in their levels of pesticide residue. Some vegetables, such as broccoli, asparagus, and onions, as well as foods with thicker peels, such as avocados, bananas, and oranges, have relatively low levels of pesticides (apart from the skin/peel) compared to other fruits and vegetables. Be aware that some vegetables and fruit contain large amounts of pesticide. Each year the Environmental Working Group releases their list of the "Dirty Dozen" fruits and vegetables and rates fruits and vegetables from worst to best. You can check it out online at www.ewg.org.

When organic vegetables or fruit that you want are not available, ask your grocer to get them. You can also look for small-operation farmers in your area and check out farmers markets in season. Many small farms can't afford to use as many chemicals in farming as large commercial farms do. Another option is to order organic produce by mail.

Avoid the "Dirty Dozen"

If you can't afford to purchase all organic produce, you could still avoid the worst pesticide-sprayed offenders by buying only organically grown produce for the top-contaminated list. (Do keep in mind, though, that this choice will not help the plight of farmworkers who fall ill and die of cancer and other diseases at a much higher percentage than the average person.) The nonprofit research organization Environmental Working Group reports periodically on health risks posed by pesticides in produce. The group says you can cut your pesticide exposure by almost 90 percent simply by avoiding the top twelve conventionally grown fruits and vegetables that have been found to be the most contaminated. It has been found that eating the twelve most contaminated fruits and vegetables will expose a person to about fourteen pesticides per day, on average. Eating the twelve least contaminated will expose a person to less than two pesticides per day. The list changes each year. To get the current ratings, got to www.ewg.org.

The Dirty Dozen List (as of 2011)[10]

1. *Apples.* Like peaches, apples are typically grown with poisons to kill a variety of pests, from fungi to insects. Tests have found forty-two different pesticides as residue on apples. Scrubbing and peeling don't eliminate chemical residues that are systemic.

2. *Celery* has no protective skin, which makes it almost impossible to wash off the chemicals (sixty-four of them!) that are used on crops.

3. *Strawberries.* If you buy strawberries, especially out of season, they're most likely imported from countries that have less stringent regulations for pesticide use; fifty-nine pesticides have been detected in residue on strawberries.

4. *Peaches.* Multiple pesticides (as many as sixty-two of them) are regularly applied to the delicate skins of this fruit in conventional orchards.

5. *Spinach.* Spinach can be contaminated with as many as forty-eight different pesticides, making it one of the most polluted green leafy vegetables.

6. *Nectarines (imported).* With thirty-three different types of pesticides found on nectarines, they rank up there with apples and peaches among the dirtiest tree fruit.

7. *Grapes*, especially imported grapes, run a much greater risk of contamination than those grown domestically. Vineyards may be sprayed with various pesticides during different growing periods of the grape, and no amount of washing or peeling will eliminate contamination because of the grape's thin skin. Remember, wine is made from grapes, which testing shows can harbor as

many as thirty-four different pesticides. (Purchase only organic wine.)

8. *Sweet bell peppers* have thin skins that don't offer much of a barrier to pesticides. They're often heavily sprayed with insecticides. Tests have found forty-nine different pesticides on sweet bell peppers.

9. *Potatoes.* Commercially farmed potatoes are some of the most pesticide-contaminated vegetables. Also, chlorpropham (CIPC), the most widely used sprout inhibitor, is applied directly to potatoes to prevent sprouting. One animal study found that CIPC had a cytolytic effect (dissolution or destruction of a cell) and reduced intracellular ATP and potassium levels along with causing an alteration in metabolism. (ATP is the energy fuel that powers our cells.)[11] One study found 81 percent of the potatoes tested still contained pesticides after being washed and peeled.[12] The potato has one of the highest pesticide counts of forty-three fruits and vegetables tested, according to the Environmental Working Group. Doesn't this make you think twice before ordering french fries?[13]

10. *Blueberries* (domestic) are treated with as many as fifty-two pesticides, making them one of the dirtiest berries on the market. A friend recently stopped by the road to pick some blueberries. A woman nearby told him that they would come by and spray all the berries in a few weeks before they were picked. She said that when they sprayed the year before, all her goldfish died, but that it didn't hurt her. Sadly, her belief is far from truth; these chemicals hurt everyone.

11. *Lettuce.* Fifty-one different pesticides have been found on lettuce including known or probable carcinogens, suspected hormone disruptors, neurotoxins, developmental or reproductive toxins, and honeybee toxins.[14]

12. *Kale/collard greens.* Traditionally, kale is known as a hardy vegetable that rarely suffers from pests and disease, but it was found to have high amounts of pesticide residue when tested in 2010. In 2011, collard leaves joined the list with kale.

The Clean Fifteen Food List (as of 2011)[15]

"The Clean Fifteen" harbored little to no traces of pesticides and is safe to consume in nonorganic form. The list includes:

- Onions
- Sweet corn
- Pineapples
- Avocado
- Asparagus
- Sweet peas
- Mangoes
- Eggplant
- Cantaloupe (domestic)
- Kiwi
- Cabbage
- Watermelon
- Sweet potatoes
- Grapefruit
- Mushrooms

COMPLETELY AVOID IRRADIATED FOODS

Nonorganic vegetables, meats, and other products have been irradiated for years. Irradiation kills insects and other bugs that may have crawled into foods before being shipped to the grocery store. From apples to zucchini, produce is routinely irradiated. It may seem that food irradiation to kill bacteria and bugs on nonorganic vegetables and meat should be beneficial. Most people would think that spinach irradiated to kill salmonella is happy spinach, right? Not necessarily.

Here's what's really going on. In order to kill all these insects, bacteria, fungus, and mold, and to give food a longer shelf life, food is exposed to radiation in very high levels. In the United States this practice began in the 1960s with the irradiation of wheat and white potatoes. Since then the FDA has approved a steady stream of foods for irradiation: in the 1980s, spices and seasonings, pork, fresh fruit, and dried and dehydrated substances were approved; in 1990, poultry; and in 1997, red meat was approved.[16]

Irradiation has been shown to produce chromosome damage. Studies performed with children in Hyderabad, India, by the National Institute of Nutrition at the Council of Medical Research showed chromosome damage after being fed freshly irradiated wheat for six weeks. Other children who were fed a similar diet that was not irradiated did not show chromosome damage. The condition gradually reversed when the children were taken off the irradiated diet.[17]

Irradiation also causes nutrient destruction. It destroys essential vitamins and minerals, including vitamin A; thiamine; vitamins B_2, B_3, B_6, and B_{12}; folic acid; and vitamins C, E, and K. Amino acid and essential fatty acid content may also be harmed. A 20 to 80 percent loss of these nutrients is common. Also, irradiation kills friendly bacteria and enzymes, rendering the food "dead" and useless to the body—the opposite of a living foods diet. And it can generate harmful by-products such as free radicals, which are toxins that can damage cells, and harmful chemicals known as *radiolytic products*, including formaldehyde and benzene.[18]

The answer to food-borne illnesses is not irradiation; the answer is stopping the overuse of pesticides, adopting sustainable organic farming practices, transforming overcrowded factory-farm animal lots to humane sanitary farms, and ensuring more sanitary conditions in food-processing plants.

The only good thing is that in the United States, food growers and manufacturers must put the irradiation symbol on the label that the food is irradiated, so avoidance of irradiated foods is possible if one shops carefully. Since 1986, all irradiated products must carry the international symbol called a *radura,* which is a flower within a circle. But it is similar to the symbol for the Environmental Protection Agency. Whenever you see this radura symbol (stylized flower), complain to your supermarket manager. However, if you eat out at a restaurant, you will not know when you're eating irradiated food, since they are not obliged to reveal that information to their customers. You can ask the server or manager, but they may not know. Some restaurants refuse to serve irradiated food, while others serve it regularly.

SAY NO TO GMO

What do tortilla chips, soy milk, and canola oil have in common? They're all made from the top GMO crops in North America.

Of the more than fifty genetically modified (GM) plant varieties that have been examined and approved for human consumption, the majority of them are modified for herbicide tolerance and pest tolerance[19]—for example, tomatoes and cantaloupes have modified ripening characteristics; soybeans and sugar beets are resistant to herbicides; and corn and cotton plants have increased resistance to insect pests.

There are other foods to watch for and buy only organic. Rice is modified to boost its vitamin A levels. Sugar cane is genetically modified to resist pesticides. A large percentage of sweeteners used in processed food actually comes from corn, not sugar cane or beets, and corn is one of the biggest GM crops in America. Beets were recently approved as a GM crop. GM papayas now make up about three quarters of the total Hawaiian papaya crop. Meat and dairy products often come from animals that have been fed or injected with GM products, which is why it's very important to purchase only pasture-fed, organically raised animal products. Genetically modified peas have created immune responses in mice, suggesting that they could also create serious allergic reactions in people. Peas had a gene inserted from kidney beans, which creates a protein that acts as a pesticide.[20] Many vegetable oils and margarines used in restaurants and in processed foods and salad dressings are made from soy, corn, canola, or cottonseed. Unless these oils specifically say "Non-GMO" or "organic," they are probably genetically modified.

When trying to avoid the top GM crops, you'll need to watch out for maltodextrin, soy lecithin, soy oil, textured vegetable protein (soy), canola oil, corn products, and high-fructose corn syrup. Other GM crops to avoid include some varieties of zucchini, crookneck squash, papayas from Hawaii, aspartame (NutraSweet), and milk containing rbGH, rennet (containing genetically modified enzymes) used to make hard cheeses. Many of these products you would not want anyway, but when it comes to these foods, unless you buy organically grown, it's quite probable you'll be eating genetically modified food. And that should cause you great concern.

Even vitamin supplements may be genetically modified or contain GM material. For example, vitamin C is often made from corn (look for "non-corn source" on the label), and vitamin E is usually made from soy. Vitamins A, B_2, B_6, B_{12}, D, and K may have fillers derived from GM corn sources, such as starch, glucose, and maltodextrin.[21]

This is precisely the reason for purchasing only high-quality vitamins from reliable sources that use organic materials.

We must become informed consumers and careful shoppers. We can look at the labels of packaged products to see if they contain corn flour or cornmeal, soy flour, cornstarch, textured vegetable protein, corn syrup, or modified food starch. Check labels of soy sauce, tofu, soy beverages, soy protein isolate, soy milk, soy ice cream, soy cheese, margarine, and soy lecithin, among dozens of other products. If it doesn't say organic or non-GMO, don't buy it; the chances are strong that they are GMO. To shop smart, see the Non-GMO Shopping Guide, created by the Institute for Responsible Technology, at www.nongmoshoppingguide.com.

When we refuse to buy GMO products, we will also help to reduce pollution. A variety of noxious gases are polluting our world, and nitrous oxide (N_2O) makes up 10 percent of them. This gas is three hundred times more destructive than CO_2 and has the ability to remain in the atmosphere almost permanently. Two-thirds of this gas emission comes from nitrate fertilizers used on genetically modified industrial farms. The largest GMO crops that utilize them are those grown with billions of tons of pesticides for factory farms and feedlots.[22]

Currently the FDA does not require that foods be labeled GMO. But without protective labeling, we will not know when we are buying them because GM foods look just like non-GMO foods. And unsuspecting consumers are eating products that have the potential to damage their health. The only way to avoid GMO foods is by becoming aware of which foods are genetically engineered and what products are made from them, and purchasing only organic foods and products made from those foods. Some estimates reveal that as many as thirty thousand different products on grocery store shelves are genetically modified, which is largely because many processed foods contain some form of soy.

Chapter 6

Beyond the Weekend: How to Keep Losing Weight and Feeling Great

AFTER YOUR WEEKEND of juicing you might be tempted to return to your regular eating habits. Instead of giving in to this temptation, I hope you'll stop and create a plan for how you'll eat smarter and healthier to build on the healthy jump start your weekend program has begun. I've even provided a menu plan and recipes in this book to help you extend your healthy eating for a full two weeks. You'll also find a list of foods to eat and foods to avoid in Appendix B. You can use this as your guideline as you embark on a new lifestyle of healthier food choices.

But even with menus, recipes, and food lists, you still need to think about how to choose the best products for a lifestyle of healthy eating and maintaining your weight. All animal products are not the same; neither are vegetables and fruit, nor anything else on the list in Appendix B for that matter. The "healthy food" issue is where the eating programs in my Juice Lady books differ from many other diet books or weight-loss programs. As I said in chapter 1, *The Juice Lady's Weekend Weight-Loss Diet* is a weight-loss program on a mission. The mission is to help you get *healthier* and thinner, not just thinner. And I want this mission to continue long after the weekend is over. That's why I'm about to build upon the key information about shopping for groceries that I provided in the last chapter. It's been said that knowledge is power, so the more you understand the difference between healthy and unhealthy foods, the more empowered you will be to make healthy food choices for a lifetime.

ANIMAL PROTEIN

Quality lean protein is important for your health and weight management. It stimulates the production of glucagon, a hormone that functions opposite insulin. Glucagon stabilizes blood sugar levels and provides brain fuel by signaling the body to release stored energy. When synchronized, insulin and glucagon create a stable hormonal system.

When choosing animal protein, opt for grass-fed (also called pastured) beef, lamb, buffalo, and poultry products whenever possible. You will get healthier meat compared with commercial products—meat that has more "good" fats and fewer unhealthy ones. For example, meat from grass-fed animals has two to four times more omega-3 fatty acids than meat from grain-fed animals. This meat is also richer in antioxidants, including vitamin E, beta-carotene, and vitamin C. Furthermore, pastured meat doesn't have traces of hormones, antibiotics, or other drugs. And it has appreciable amounts of CLA (conjugated linoleic acid), three to five times more than products from animals fed conventional diets.[1] Listen up! Studies have shown CLA to promote weight loss. It's a naturally occurring fatty acid found in animal and dairy fats such as beef, lamb, dairy products, poultry, and eggs. Recent studies have also shown possible health benefits from CLA, such as inhibiting tumor formation, maintaining healthy blood vessels, and normalizing metabolism of glucose.[2]

If you can't find grass-fed meat, do shop for free-range or, at the very least, antibiotic-free beef, dairy, lamb, buffalo, and poultry. The growth hormones injected into factory-farmed animals cause them to gain weight. After all, fattening animals quickly to get them to market means more dollars for vendors. But what does it mean for us? These hormones are not healthful; they are even harmful to us. Natural foods markets such as Whole Foods, Wild Oats, co-ops, and many independent health food markets as well as local farmers have pastured or naturally raised beef, lamb, buffalo, and poultry.

Keep in mind that you can get too much animal protein, which is taxing for the kidneys and can contribute to overacidity in the system. That is why it's best to limit portion sizes to between 4 and 6 ounces, with women eating no more than 4 ounces.

Wise Up About Red Meat

Not all red meat is created equal. In addition to being higher in omega-3 fats and CLA, meat from grass-fed animals is also higher in vitamin E. In fact, studies show the meat from pastured cattle is four times higher in vitamin E than meat from feedlot cattle and, interestingly, almost twice as high as the meat from feedlot cattle given vitamin E supplements. That's beneficial, in that vitamin E is linked with a lower risk of heart disease and cancer.[3]

Grass-fed beef is also lower in total fat and particularly the saturated fats linked to heart disease. It's also higher in beta-carotene, the B vitamins thiamine and riboflavin, and the minerals calcium, magnesium, and potassium.

A team of scientists from the USDA compared grass-fed lambs with lambs fed grain in a feedlot. They found that lambs grazing on pasture had 14 percent less fat and about 8 percent more protein compared to grain-fed lamb. And check this out! Meat from sheep raised on pasture has shown twice as much lutein (carotene) as meat from grain-fed sheep. Lutein reduces the risk of cataracts and macular degeneration (a leading cause of blindness) and may also help prevent breast and colon cancer.[4]

PASTURED POULTRY VERSUS FREE-RANGE OR COMMERCIAL FOWL

Pasture-raised poultry are far healthier than commercial-raised fowl. Pastured poultry are chickens, turkey, ducks, and geese that are raised in bottomless cages or pens outside or on grass where they can peck and scratch at the ground and hunt for bugs and seeds along with their grain. They breathe fresh air and roam in the sun. Their manure is spread over wide areas of pasture as they are moved, which is good for the soil as well as the birds.

Sometimes they are mistakenly called free-range chickens, but free-range birds are still kept in confinement; they are just allowed to roam inside their buildings, which are often very crowded so "roaming" is not really possible.

Commercially raised factory farm birds fare the worst. They are housed in confinement with their feet standing in their own manure from birth to death. They do not get the benefits of fresh air and sunshine or the grass, seeds, and bugs of the pasture they are meant to eat. They are drugged and sick most of their lives.

When you choose pasture-raised chicken, you avoid the following:

- *Hormones, antibiotics, and drugs.* There is growing concern that hormone and drug residues in muscle meats, eggs, and milk might be harmful to human health and the environment. There may be immunological effects and cancer risks for consumers.[5]

- *Arsenic.* Commercial poultry are often fed trace amounts of arsenic in their feed to stimulate their appetites. Traces of arsenic can be found in the meat we buy.[6]

EGGS FROM PASTURED HENS

Eggs contain all eight essential amino acids and are a rich source of essential fatty acids, especially when raised on pasture. They also contain considerably more lecithin (a fat emulsifier) than cholesterol. Additionally, eggs from hens bred outdoors have four to six times more vitamin D than eggs from hens bred in confinement.[7] Pastured hens are exposed to direct sunlight, which is converted to vitamin D and passed on to the eggs. And the eggs are rich in sulfur and glutathione.

Look for eggs from chickens that are raised cage-free on pasture, without hormones, and fed an organic diet that includes green grass. When chickens are housed indoors and deprived of greens, their eggs become low in good fats.

For organic pastured eggs, look to co-ops and natural food markets; also seek out local producers, farmers, and homesteaders who pasture their poultry or let them roam free.

Lab Tests on Eggs From Pastured Chickens

Mother Earth News collected samples from fourteen pastured chicken flocks across the country and had them tested at an accredited laboratory. The results were compared to official USDA data for commercial eggs. Results showed the pastured eggs contained an astounding:

- One-third less cholesterol than commercial eggs
- One-fourth less saturated fat
- Two-thirds more vitamin A
- Two times more omega-3 fatty acids
- Seven times more beta-carotene[8]

Fish

To select the best fish, buy only wild-caught—meaning caught with a boat and hook or net. The other option is ranched or farm-raised fish, which you should avoid. Farm-raised fish are housed within small pens that are set up in the ocean or in small ponds. The fish are often kept in overcrowded conditions, which increase their risk of infection and disease. Instead of being allowed to find their own natural food sources (other fish and krill), they're fed dried food pellets made up of fish oil, fish meal containing concentrations of toxins, chicken feces, corn meal, soy, genetically modified canola oil, and other fish. The dried food pellets are often contaminated with such cancer-causing agents as PCBs, dioxins, and even flame-retardants. This creates a very unnatural environment, which yields unhealthy fish. In fact, because their flesh looks anemic, these fish are given artificial colorings in their food to get the same coloration back that wild salmon have naturally.

Because farm-raised fish are susceptible to disease due to their overcrowded living conditions, they're often given antibiotics, which become part of the flesh. Some sources say that salmon are given more antibiotics than farm animals. In contrast, wild salmon are relatively free of these substances and disease.

Farm-raised fish do not have the essential fatty acids that wild-caught fish offer and that are so important for our health. When it comes to animal fat, wild-caught fish are a good source of the healthy omega-3 fatty acids, especially coldwater fish such as salmon, mackerel, and trout. Also, the smaller the fish, the less mercury and other heavy metals that will be stored in the flesh and fat.

Fats and Oils

For decades we've have had a love-hate relationship with this food that makes so many dishes taste great. Fat gives us that feeling of satisfaction we all long for—satiety, actually—that we've had enough to eat. But that's not all. Fats play an important role in our body's health. Some fats can even help us lose weight. Unfortunately, we consume too few of the healthy fats and too many of the unhealthy man-made versions.

It's difficult to eat enough food on a low-fat diet to get the energy we need. Fat provides that energy. Essential fats such as fish oils are brain food—a deficiency can lead to numerous health and psychiatric/social problems. We need fats to absorb fat-soluble vitamins such as A, D, E, and K. But which fats are the best choices? Which fats can be harmful to our bodies? And which ones, because of their chemical processing, have the most negative impact on our health and the environment?

Since the 1950s we've been told to use vegetable oil for heart health. It looks clear and pure in a bottle on your shelf. No worries, right? Oh, so wrong. We've been led astray. Polyunsaturated oils (corn, safflower, sunflower, soy, cottonseed) are especially susceptible to oxidation because they have more than one double bond, which can be broken rather easily when exposed to heat, sunlight, and oxygen. This is why they have the greatest tendency to oxidize. This triggers inflammation, a leading cause of heart disease, and can damage blood vessels. Oxidation can happen even in the processing of these oils, and it is accelerated with heat, which they undergo in processing unless they are cold processed. The oils are then deodorized, which means that we can't smell when they are rancid. Rancid oil generates free radicals, which are produced in the processing and are one of the primary causes of oxidized cholesterol. It is oxidized cholesterol that is implicated in heart disease, not general LDL. This is the reason unsaturated fats are so dangerous. There should be a warning on every label so consumers can make an educated purchase, but then that would curtail profits.

Oxidized oils also damage cells, causing inflammation.

Inflammation produces insulin resistance, and insulin resistance produces weight gain. Weight gain generates inflammatory cytokines, leading to more insulin resistance and more weight gain. It becomes a frustrating cycle of gaining more and more weight.

When people eat foods prepared with processed vegetable oils—margarine, french fries, fried food, nonfat dried milk, powdered or liquid coffee creamer, many salad dressings, crackers, cookies, chips, and a plethora of processed and convenience foods—they eat a high quantity of oxidized (rancid) oil. This sets up the body for disease.

To help you choose the very best oils and fats, here's your shopping guide for the healthiest fats and oils, along with the ones to avoid. I've also included the smoke point of the oils recommended, which is the point at which fat breaks down, starts to smoke, and gives off an odor, accelerating the oxidation of these oils.

Coconut oil. Choose only organic virgin coconut oil, which means it has been made by a traditional method that does not involve high heat or harmful chemicals. It won't oxidize (turn rancid) as easily because it doesn't have the double bonds that make polyunsaturated oils most vulnerable to oxidation. It has a longer shelf life (about two years) than most oils and does not need to be refrigerated. It has been a staple cooking oil for thousands of years in tropical climates. It is white when solid, creamy colored when liquid.

Many commercial-grade coconut oils are made from copra, which means the dried kernel (meat) of the coconut. If standard copra is used as a starting material, the unrefined coconut oil extracted from copra is not suitable for human consumption and must be refined. This is because most copra is dried under the sun in the open air in very unsanitary conditions where it's exposed to insects and molds. Though producers may start with organic coconuts and even label their coconut oil organic, the end product of some brands is refined, bleached, and deodorized oil. High heat and chemical solvents are usually used in this process. If you select virgin coconut oil made by hand the old-fashioned way, you will immediately notice the difference in taste, smell, and texture from oil made with standard copra. The traditionally made oil, which is known as virgin coconut oil, is far superior in every way. You will pay more for this oil, but it's well worth it.

Research has shown that coconut oil can help you lose weight—the body likes to burn its medium-chain fatty acids rather than store them as it does long-chain fatty acids that dominate many other oils.[9] It has a "thermogenic effect," meaning it raises body temperature, thus boosting energy and metabolic rate and promoting weight loss. It has also been shown in a university study to kill yeasts, even *Candida albicans*.[10] Coconut oil is great for medium-heat cooking (smoke point of 350 degrees). It has no cholesterol, which some have claimed. And it tastes great on popcorn.

Olive oil is an outstanding monounsaturated fat. A tablespoon of extra-virgin olive oil contains 11 grams of monounsaturated fat, 2 grams of saturated fat, and 1 gram of polyunsaturated fat. An ancient oil dating back to biblical times, it was used for cooking and healing. It is more shelf stable than polyunsaturated oils. The most flavorful, healthful and eco-friendly varieties are extra-virgin organic oils that are cold-pressed or expeller-pressed. These are produced without chemical solvents such as hexane and high heat. High-quality olive oil stands out also as an antioxidant that is a free-radical fighter.

Olive oil is great for salad dressings, cold foods, and low-heat cooking such as light sautéing. Extra-virgin olive oil has a smoke point of 305–320 degrees. Other monounsaturated oils such as avocado and almond oil are better suited for higher-heat cooking.

Completely avoid the less expensive, chemically derived version called olive pomace oil—the last dregs of the olive oil pressing process, extracted by petroleum solvents such as hexane.

Almond oil is monounsaturated oil that is extracted from the almond and has a distinctively nutty flavor. It is typically used as an ingredient in salad dressings, sauces, mayonnaise, and desserts. Unlike almond extract, almond oil is not concentrated enough to provide a strong almond taste. It is suited for high-heat cooking and baking with a smoke point of 420 degrees. Many toxic pesticides and herbicides are used on almond trees; therefore, choose only organic cold-pressed or expeller-pressed almond oil.

Avocado oil is extracted from the avocado by pressing the flesh, not the seed. It is often compared to olive oil because the oils are similar in composition, but avocado oil has a much higher smoke point of 520 degrees and is good for high-heat cooking and baking. High-quality avocado oil has a distinct green color due to its chlorophyll content. It also has a characteristic avocado flavor, depending on how the oil has been processed and handled and the quality of the avocados used. Avocado oil is fairly shelf stable and does not oxidize easily. Choose cold-pressed or expeller-pressed avocado oil. Avoid chemically processed oil altogether.

Rice bran oil is extracted from the germ and inner husk of rice. It is dominantly monounsaturated. A tablespoon contains 7 grams of monounsaturated fat, 3 grams of saturated fat, and 5 grams of polyunsaturated fat. It contains healthful phytochemicals such as beta-sitosterol, which can reduce the absorption of cholesterol, and alpha-linoleic acid, which can increase essential fatty acid concentration.

Rice bran oil has a mild taste and is popular in Asian cuisine because of its suitability for high-temperature cooking such as stir-frying, with a smoke point of 490 degrees. It is said to be the secret of good tempura. Rice bran oil also contains components of vitamin E that may benefit health and prevent rancidity. Look for organic, cold-pressed or expeller-pressed oil.

Peanut oil (unrefined) has a smoke point of 320 degrees, which makes it good for only low-heat cooking. Refined peanut oil has a much higher smoke point but is not recommended because of being refined. Peanut oil contains 48 percent monounsaturated fat, 18 percent saturated fat, and 34 percent polyunsaturated fat. Like olive oil, peanut oil is relatively stable and, therefore, appropriate for stir-fry. But the high percentage of omega-6 fatty acids it contains presents a potential problem since the American diet contains far too much omega-6 already and not enough omega-3 fats. Limit your use of peanut oil or avoid it altogether. Peanuts are grown underground and known to absorb toxins from the soil, so choose only organic, cold-pressed or expeller-pressed oil.

Sesame oil contains 42 percent monounsaturated fat, 15 percent saturated fat, and 43 percent polyunsaturated fat. It has been used for thousands of years in Asian culture. Sesame oil is similar in composition to peanut oil. The high percentage of omega-6 fats indicates that it should be used only occasionally in small quantities. Hexane is typically used to extract oil from the seeds, so choose only cold-pressed or expeller-pressed oil, and always refrigerate it. Organic is better, but pesticide residues are minor in nonorganic sesame seeds and oils.

Macadamia nut oil is expressed from the meat of the macadamia. Native to Australia, the oil contains approximately 60 percent monounsaturated fat, about 20 percent saturated fat, and 20 percent polyunsaturated fat. Some varieties contain roughly equal omega-6s and omega-3s. It is very shelf stable due to its low polyunsaturated fat content. It has a smoke point of 410 degrees, making it suitable for higher-heat cooking. Few pesticides are used on these nuts, so organic oil is not necessary. But choose only cold-pressed or expeller-pressed oil because the highest concentration of hexane residue was found in macadamia nut oil in a study that tested 41 samples of vegetable, fruit, and nut oils.[11]

Butter. Purchase organic butter from grass-fed cows. It has more cancer-fighting conjugated linoleic acid (CLA), vitamin E, beta-carotene, and omega-3 fatty acids than butter from cows raised on factory farms or that have limited access to pasture. A 2006 study showed that the cows who ate the most fresh grass had the softer the butter. Cows that eat only grass have the softest butterfat of all.[12]

Butter is dominated by short- and medium-chain fatty acids. It's a healthier choice than margarine or most other vegetable spreads, with the exception of coconut oil and olive oil spreads. Butter is a rich source of vitamins A, E, K, and D. It also has appreciable amounts of butyric acid, which is used by the colon as an energy source, and lauric acid, a medium-chain fatty acid that is a potent antimicrobial and antifungal substance. Butter from grass-fed cows also contains CLA, which gives excellent protection against cancer and helps us lose weight. Because living grass is richer in vitamins E, A, and beta-carotene than stored hay or standard diets for dairy cows, butter from dairy cows grazing on fresh pasture is also richer in these important nutrients. The naturally golden color of grass-fed butter is a good indication of its superior nutritional value.[13]

Butter is suited for medium-heat cooking with a smoke point of 350 degrees. Ghee, which is clarified butter, has a smoke point between 375 and 485 degrees and is good for medium to high-heat cooking.

AVOID THESE COMPLETELY

Polyunsaturated oils. In their natural state, as found in nuts, vegetables, and seeds, polyunsaturated fats are healthy. But when they are processed into oil, they oxidize easily and do more harm than good. In the past half century, the ratio of omega-6 fats, from polyunsaturated oils (corn, safflower, sunflower, cottonseed, and soybean oils), to omega-3 fats has changed in the Western diet from 2:1 to 14 to 25:1, which promotes inflammation, weight gain, depression, and immune system dysfunction. Our diets now include too few omega-3s, which are found primarily in fish, fish oil, seafood, grass-fed meat and dairy, walnuts, flax, hemp, and chia seeds, and in smaller amounts in vegetables, whole grains, and beans.

Canola oil is a monounsaturated fat, as is olive oil, which means it contains only one double bond, so technically it could be used for salad dressings, cold food preparation, and low-temperature cooking. But there's a major reason not to use it: most canola oil comes from GM crops. Researchers at the University of Florida in Gainesville found trans fat levels as high as 4.6 percent in processed canola oil.[14]

Trans fats are created in the process of hydrogenating oils and should be avoided completely. The consumption of trans fats increases the risk of coronary heart disease. Commercially baked goods such as crackers, cookies, cakes, muffins, and many fried foods, such as doughnuts and french fries, may contain trans fats. Mainstream shortenings and some margarine can be high in trans fat.

Margarine and butter replacement spreads. Margarine is made from different types of oils mixed with emulsifiers, vitamins, coloring, flavoring, and other ingredients. The oils often are hydrogenated—a process used to solidify them, making the margarine solid and spreadable. The *New York Times* says, "A new report by Harvard researchers says a fat [trans fat] in margarine and other processed foods could be responsible for 30,000 of the nation's annual deaths from heart disease."[15] When it comes to natural spreads that are substitutes for butter, read labels; know what oils are used. An olive oil or coconut oil spread would be fine, but anything made with polyunsaturated oils or canola oil (unless it specifically says non-GMO) should be avoided.

Salt. Choose only Celtic sea salt or gray salt. Whole sea salt has a mineral profile that is similar to our blood. Regular table salt is highly refined sodium chloride that usually contains additives to make it pour easily. When salt is processed, minerals are removed. Then, anti-caking chemicals such as potassium oxide or aluminum calcium silicate, iodine, and dextrose (sugar) are added to make table salt. Eat salt sparingly, even Celtic or gray salt. It causes the body to retain water.

Sugar—all types. Most of the sugar we eat is disguised in sodas and other drinks, desserts, boxed cereals, energy bars, packaged foods, snacks, and yogurt. Much of it is high-fructose corn syrup, which is used to sweeten everything from crackers, tomato sauces, ketchup, sodas, processed meats, and even some health food products. It's used primarily because it's cheap. But many health professionals attribute it to the increase in obesity, metabolic syndrome, diabetes, certain cancers, and heart disease. The more you avoid sugar, the less you will crave it. And you'll lose weight!

Check out the website www.sugarshock.com. You'll learn about journalist Connie Bennett's journey to a changed life by avoiding sugar. She suffered from dozens of debilitating symptoms for years. Finally a doctor connected her condition to overeating processed carbohydrates and sweets, which included her favorites—red licorice, chocolate, and hard candy.

All of these sugar sources need to be avoided: high-fructose corn syrup, sucrose (white sugar—another big GMO product), brown sugar, honey, dextrin (a complex sugar molecule, left over from enzyme action on starch), sugar alcohols such as sorbitol and manitol, xylitol (choose only organic from birch trees—much of the xylitol on the market is made from by-products of the wood pulp industry or from cane pulp, seed hulls, or corn husk), cane juice, sucanat, and molasses.

Artificial sweeteners. For the sake of your health, not just your weight, completely avoid all artificial sweeteners, which can cause a host of health problems. And if you think they're helping you lose weight, take a look at the research. People on sugar substitutes actually gain more weight than those using sugar.[16] And using sugar is a very bad choice for your weight as well as your health.

Check out the movie *Sweet Misery* for an eye-opening report on aspartame (NutraSweet). Dr. Woodrow C. Monte says, "Methanol [one of the breakdown products of aspartame] is considered a toxicant. The ingestion of two teaspoons is considered lethal in humans."[17] Long-term use can create a ticking time bomb for a large array of neurological illnesses, including (but not limited to) brain cancer, Lou Gehrig's disease, Graves' disease, chronic fatigue syndrome, multiple sclerosis (MS), and epilepsy.[18]

James Turner, chairman of Citizens for Health, has declared that the FDA should review their approval of Splenda based on a study of sucralose that reveals shocking new information about the potential harmful effects of this artificial sweetener on humans. Hundreds of consumers have complained about side effects from using Splenda. Turner went on to say that the study, published in the *Journal of Toxicology and Environmental Health*, confirms that the chemicals in the little yellow packets "should carry a big red warning label." According to a press release from the Citizens for Health, the study found that "Splenda reduces the amount of good bacteria in the intestines by 50%, increases the pH level in the intestines, contributes to increases in body weight, and affects the P-glycoprotein (P-gp) in the body in such a way that crucial health-related drugs could be rejected."[19] The study is clear that this sweetener can also cause you to gain weight!

High-Fructose Corn Syrup Makes Your Brain Crave Food

The average American now consumes 145 pounds of high-fructose corn syrup per year (a corn sweetener found in most sodas and many processed foods). It's amazing everyone is not obese. New research proves exactly how high-fructose corn syrup bypasses normal energy balance systems in the body, causing the brain to want more food because it never really registers the calories of the high-fructose corn syrup.[20] There is also research indicating that high-fructose corn syrup turns on gene signaling that promotes fat formation and fat accumulation, which is likely to result in obesity, insulin resistance, and type 2 diabetes.[21]

Sweeteners to use sparingly include agave syrup, brown rice syrup, and pure maple syrup. Raw honey is also acceptable if used sparingly. I recommend stevia as the best sweetener to use.

Take Supplements for Weight Management

Multivitamins

When you're cutting back on food in general, and certain foods such as fruit and grains in particular, it's important to fill in the gaps with a good multivitamin capsule. Be aware that not all supplements are high quality. You will pay a little more for a natural high-quality supplement, but it's worth it.

Enzyme supplements

Digestive enzymes can play a big part in weight control. A lack of enzymes is a hidden factor in obesity. Enzymes are essential for supporting healthy weight loss. Lipase is an enzyme that is abundant in raw foods, and since very few of us have a diet rich in raw foods, we lack sufficient amounts to digest normal amounts of fat in our diets. When we eat diets rich in fat but low in enzyme-rich raw food, our bodies can't burn this extra fat as efficiently or turn it into energy. When we have enough lipase, our bodies are able to break down and utilize the fat. Without this vital enzyme, fat accumulates and is stored in arteries, organs, capillaries, and, of course, fat cells. You will see it pack onto your hips, buttocks, stomach, and thighs.

Protease is a vital enzyme for breaking down proteins and

eliminating toxins. If your body is storing toxins, it becomes more difficult to burn fat—fat cells are where your body stores excess toxins. When you do burn fat, toxins are released back into your system, which can cause water retention and bloating. So a diet rich in protease, or enzyme supplementation, will help to eliminate toxins, which is why these two enzymes are so important when you are losing weight.

Amylase is an enzyme that breaks starch down into sugar. Amylase is present in human saliva—the mouth is where the chemical process of digestion begins. Amylase assists in the digestion of starches and carbohydrates and, when combined with the other enzymes, supports overall digestion. It also serves as a glucose balancer.

Calcium

One study found that a diet consisting mainly of high-calcium foods resulted in an average weight loss of 24.6 pounds in sixteen weeks.[22] This is greater than the average weight loss in one year in trials using weight-loss drugs. According to the *Journal of the American College of Nutrition*, fifty-four young women participated in a two-year study; those with the highest intakes of calcium lost the most weight and body fat on weight-control programs, regardless of exercise level.[23] Other peer-reviewed trials continue to indicate that high-calcium diets are associated with lower body weight. In another study, researchers estimated that only 1,000 milligrams of additional calcium intake daily resulted in a 17.6-pound difference in body weight.[24] (See Appendix A for calcium recommendations.)

Vitamin D

A University of Minnesota study has found that higher levels of vitamin D on a low-calorie diet may help people lose more weight, especially around the abdomen. The study found that subjects lost a quarter to a half pound more fat when their vitamin D level was increased.[25] (See Appendix A for vitamin D recommendations.)

5-hydroxytryptophan (5-HTP)

5-HTP is the immediate precursor to serotonin and has been studied in the treatment of obesity. One study concluded that 5-HTP reduced the total number of daily calories without a conscience effort to lose weight by any of the female participants. Average weight loss in this particular study was 3 pounds over the course of five weeks.[26] A second study involved a six-week period without dietary restriction and the second six weeks with the addition of a 1,200-calorie diet. There was a marked increase in weight loss of participants taking the supplement versus those given a placebo. The average weight loss was 10.3 pounds for the supplement group and 2.28 pounds for the placebo group. The conclusion was that 5-HTP's action on the satiety center of the brain caused users to eat fewer calories.[27] Also, 5-HTP helps some individuals alleviate insomnia. And 5-HTP helps depression, which could reduce emotional eating due to depressed moods such as sadness, loneliness, and self-loathing.

Maca powder

Maca is an annual plant grown in Peru that produces a radish-like root. The Peruvians claim that Maca increases energy, helps depression and anemia, and improves overall memory and vitality. This powerful food is also a libido stimulant! More energy equates to more activity and burning more calories.

Inulin

Inulin is a low-glycemic, soluble fiber that assumes a gel-like consistency when exposed to water. Inulin increases satiety—the sensation of fullness. It's found in sunchokes (Jerusalem artichokes), asparagus stems, chicory root (used most often to make commercial inulin), artichoke bulb, and salsify root. This fiber cuts your craving for food. Also, the probiotic nature of inulin helps provide an environment for healthy bacteria to continue growing in the intestinal tract. A study with children published in the *Journal of Pediatrics* showed that supplements of inulin resulted in a much lower body mass index (BMI) over a one-year period.[28]

STAY FIT AND FAB WITH EXERCISE

What can ten minutes of brisk exercise do for you? A recent study indicated that ten minutes of vigorous exercise triggers metabolic changes that can last at least an hour. Further, the more fit you are, the more benefits you'll get. Researchers measured biochemical changes in the blood of a variety of people. Metabolic changes that started after ten minutes on a treadmill were still measurable sixty minutes after people cooled down.[29]

At Massachusetts General Hospital, researchers measured biochemical changes that occur during exercise. They found alterations in more than twenty different metabolites. Some of these compounds help you burn calories and fat, while others help stabilize your blood sugar. Some of the metabolites revved up during exercise, such as those involved in processing fat, while others involved with cellular stress decreased.[30]

The best way to burn fat and lose weight is now proving to be short bursts of anaerobic exercise in which you raise your heart rate up to your anaerobic threshold for twenty to thirty seconds and then recover for ninety seconds. This could be fast walking alternating with slow walking. My favorite is an interval class that incorporates both step aerobic and alternate weight-lifting exercises. This short-burst type of exercise can increase your human growth hormone (HGH) level, which helps you sleep better as well as lose weight, improve muscle tone, reduce wrinkles, and increase energy. The longer you can keep your body producing higher levels of HGH, the longer you will experience robust health and strength.[31]

What to Do if You Have Physical Limitations

Consider using a rebounder, a lymphasizer, or a swimming pool if you have physical limitations or disabilities. For my recommendations of specific products, see Appendix A.

STRETCHING, RELAXATION, AND BREATHING EXERCISES

Throughout history, many societies have devised exercises that are designed to strengthen and stretch the body while relaxing and focusing the mind. Some of these techniques have elaborate philosophies associated with them, yet the simple essence of their techniques is to stretch and relax the muscles, plus control breathing, so that more oxygen is delivered into the cells, especially the brain, thus calming and relaxing the whole body.

Stretching and relaxation exercises can increase suppleness, enhance mental and physical relaxation, and improve the quality of your sleep. Stretching is something nearly everyone can do, no matter what age or level of ability. Gentle movements, deep breathing, and long stretches are ideal methods of increasing flexibility and relaxation. The advantage of stretching is that it strengthens the nervous system and relieves stress and anxiety. It also strengthens and relaxes the skeletal, muscular, digestive, cardiovascular, and glandular systems, thus helping to calm the body and mind. The body is not overstimulated, as with more strenuous exercise, making this a good choice toward the end of the day.

Pilates

Pilates, a series of exercises designed to improve flexibility and strength through a variety of stretching and balancing movements, has become increasingly popular in the last several years. It typically gives people a longer, leaner appearance. A regular Pilates regimen results in a flatter stomach, thinner waist, and leaner thighs, as well as increased mobility in joints. Pilates helps improve strength, tone, flexibility, and balance, and makes the body less prone to injury. It reduces stress, relieves tension, and boosts energy through deep stretching. It also strengthens the back and spine. Physiotherapists recommend Pilates to those seeking rehabilitation after injuries to their limbs. Pilates is recommended for everyone—young, elderly, sedentary, those who suffer from osteoporosis, and those who are overweight.

CREATING THE BODY YOU'VE ALWAYS WANTED

Imagine yourself six months from now with flabby arms and legs, overweight, and discouraged about your appearance. You're fatigued, forgetful, depressed, and catching every "bug" that comes along. How do you feel? Now imagine yourself six months from now with good muscle tone, at or nearing your ideal weight, energetic with plenty of stamina, a positive mental attitude, and vibrant health. How do you feel this time?

The choices you make today will create the fitness and health you will have in the future and the body you will have six months from now. Taking action is key. If you continue in the same old rut, you will get more of the same, and nothing will change. It's time to get going on a new plan of action. Research indicates that people who have active lifestyles appear to have what can be called a "compelling future." This means that having a picture of a positive future can motivate you to do what is necessary to make your desired future a reality.

Here's what you can do right now. Imagine yourself six months to a year from now. We'll call this your "future self." When you see your future self clearly, imagine moving over and physically becoming that person. Now step back and look at your future self again. Ask that future self what he or she wants you to begin doing now to have a more active, healthy lifestyle that can create that future desired self. Whatever your future self says, write it down. Take a look around you. Notice several people who are older than you. Think about them one at a time. Which one is most like the person you'd like to be five, ten, fifteen, and twenty years from now? Which one is closest to living the lifestyle that you would like to have at that age? Write down the activities and health habits that person has developed.

Remember that each day you are creating one of two pictures—your best or your worst self. People who create the best possible future make continual positive decisions for fitness' sake, like juicing vegetables each day and exercising thirty minutes to an hour three or four times a week. They often use the stairs rather than an elevator and order more salads than sandwiches or pizza. They take more walks. They spend more time in positive pursuits. And they know about deferred gratification. They think about the consequences of daily decisions and how these choices steer them away from or toward their best future self.

Now cut out or draw a picture of your best future self and one of your worst future self. Underneath each picture write down the good or bad habits that would create either person. Put these pictures up where you can look at them every day. Each morning make a decision to choose activities and actions that will correspond with creating your best self. The rewards are immense. It's worth the effort. Every evening look again at the two pictures and evaluate which picture you moved toward that day by your actions.

What kind of body will you need to complete your goals and dreams? What weight should you be at to meet your goals? What level of health do you need to fulfill your destiny?

Your future is in your hands—one choice, maybe one sip of juice or bite of food at a time.

Chapter 7

The Weekend Weight-Loss Recipes

T HE JUICE RECIPES in this chapter use more vegetables than fruit, and the fruits and vegetables are mostly low glycemic. You may change any of the recipes to fit your needs. If there is something you are allergic to in a recipe, omit it or substitute another food. If you are diabetic, prediabetic, hypoglycemic, have a problem with yeast, or have cancer, you may need to omit almost all fruit, with the exception of lemons and limes. Berries and green apples are next in line as the lowest sugar fruits. And lemon is a nice addition to almost any recipe; it's also very alkaline.

Vegetable Juice Recipes for Vibrant Health

Cran-Apple Cocktail

2 organic green apples
¼–½ cup fresh or frozen (thawed) cranberries
½ lemon, peeled
1-inch-chunk ginger root
¼ cup purified water (optional)

Cut produce to fit your juicer's feed tube. Juice 1 apple first. Turn off the machine, add the cranberries, put the plunger in, then turn the machine on and juice. Follow with the lemon, ginger, and second apple.

Add water as needed. Stir and pour into a glass; drink as soon as possible. Serves 1–2.

Garlic Wonder

1 handful of parsley
1 dark green lettuce leaf such as green leaf or romaine
½ cucumber, peeled
1 garlic clove
3 carrots, scrubbed well, tops removed, ends trimmed
2 stalks celery with leaves, as desired

Roll the parsley in the lettuce leaf. Juice the cucumber, then the parsley rolled in the lettuce leaf. Add the garlic and push through the juicer with the carrots, followed by the celery. Stir and pour into a glass. Serves 1–2.

Twisted Ginger

4 carrots, scrubbed well, tops removed, ends trimmed
1 handful of parsley
1 lemon, peeled
1 apple
2-inch-chunk fresh ginger root, peeled

Cut produce to fit your juicer's feed tube. Juice ingredients and stir. Pour into a glass and drink as soon as possible. Serves 1–2.

Triple C

4 stalks organic celery with leaves, as desired
4 carrots, scrubbed well, tops removed, ends trimmed
¼ small head green cabbage

Cut produce to fit your juicer's feed tube. Juice ingredients and stir. Pour into a glass and drink as soon as possible. Serves 1–2.

Tomato and Spice

2 medium tomatoes
2 dark green leaves
2 radishes
1 small handful of parsley
1 lime or lemon, peeled if not organic
Dash of hot sauce

Cut produce to fit your juicer's feed tube. Juice ingredients and stir. Pour into a glass and drink as soon as possible. Serves 1.

Refreshing Mint Cocktail

2 stalks fennel with leaves
1 cucumber, peeled if not organic
1 stalk celery
1 green apple such as Granny Smith or Pippin
1 handful of mint
1-inch-chunk ginger root

Cut produce to fit your juicer's feed tube. Juice ingredients and stir. Pour into a glass and drink as soon as possible. Serves 1–2.

Beet, Carrot, Coconut Blast

4–5 carrots, scrubbed well, tops removed, ends trimmed
1 small beet with leaves

½–1 cup coconut milk
Dash cayenne pepper

Juice the carrots and beets. Pour into a glass and add the coconut milk and cayenne pepper. Stir. Drink as soon as possible. Serves 2.

Jícama Delight

2-inch by 4- or 5-inch-chunk of jícama, scrubbed well or peeled
½ green apple
½ cucumber, peeled if not organic
¼ daikon radish, trimmed and scrubbed
1-inch-chunk ginger root, scrubbed, peeled if old
½ lemon or lime, peeled if not organic

Cut produce to fit your juicer's feed tube. Juice ingredients and stir. Pour into a glass and drink as soon as possible. Serves 1.

Radish Surprise

5 carrots, scrubbed well, tops removed, ends trimmed
1 cucumber, peeled if not organic, or 1 large chunk of jícama
5–6 radishes
1 lemon, peeled if not organic

Cut produce to fit your juicer's feed tube. Juice all the ingredients. Stir the juice and pour into a glass. Serve at room temperature or chilled, as desired. Serves 1.

Root Veggie Medley

3–4 carrots, scrubbed well, tops removed, ends trimmed

1 cucumber, peeled if not organic

½ beet, scrubbed well, with stems and leaves

1 kohlrabi, with leaves

1 lemon, peeled if not organic

½ apple (green has less sugar)

1-inch-chunk ginger root, peeled

Cut produce to fit your juicer's feed tube. Juice all ingredients and stir. Pour into a glass and drink as soon as possible. Serves 1–2.

South of the Border Cocktail

1 medium tomato

1 cucumber, peeled if not organic

1 handful of cilantro

1 lime, peeled if not organic

Dash of hot sauce (optional)

Cut produce to fit your juicer's feed tube. Juice ingredients and stir. Pour into a glass and drink as soon as possible. Serves 1.

You Are Loved Cocktail

3 carrots, scrubbed well, tops removed, ends trimmed

2 celery stalks, with leaves

1 cucumber, peeled if not organic

1 handful of spinach

1 lemon, peeled if not organic

½ beet, scrubbed well, with stems and leaves

Cut produce to fit your juicer's feed tube. Juice all ingredients and stir. Pour into a glass and drink as soon as possible. Serves 1–2.

Springtime Tonic

1 tomato
1 cucumber, peeled if not organic
8 asparagus stems
Handful of wild greens
1 lemon, peeled if not organic

Cut produce to fit your juicer's feed tube. Juice all ingredients and stir. Pour into a glass and drink as soon as possible. Serves 1–2.

The Ginger Hopper With a Twist

5 medium carrots, scrubbed well, tops removed, ends trimmed
1 green apple
1-inch-chunk fresh ginger root, peeled
½ lemon, peeled if not organic

Cut produce to fit your juicer's feed tube. Juice ingredients and stir. Pour into a glass and drink as soon as possible. Serves 1.

Pink Morning

1 large pink grapefruit, peeled
½ green apple
1-inch-chunk fresh ginger root, peeled

Cut produce to fit your juicer's feed tube. Juice

ingredients and stir. Pour into a glass and drink as soon as possible. Serves 1.

Tomato Florentine

2 tomatoes
4–5 sprigs of basil
1 large handful of spinach
1 lemon, peeled if not organic

Juice one tomato. Wrap the basil in several spinach leaves. Turn off the machine and add the spinach and basil. Turn the machine back on and gently tap to juice them. Juice the remaining tomato and lemon. Stir juice, pour in a glass and drink as soon as possible. Serves 1.

Veggie Time Cocktail

4 carrots, scrubbed well, tops removed, ends trimmed
1 handful of rapini or other dark greens
1 lemon, peeled if not organic
2-inch-chunk jícama, scrubbed or peeled if not organic
1 handful of watercress
1 garlic clove

Cut produce to fit your juicer's feed tube. Juice ingredients and stir. Pour into a glass and drink as soon as possible. Serves 1–2.

Waldorf Twist

1 green apple
3 stalks organic celery with leaves
1 lemon, peeled if not organic

Cut produce to fit your juicer's feed tube. Juice ingredients and stir. Pour into a glass and drink as soon as possible. Serves 1.

GREEN JUICES

Green Refresher

1 medium to large organic cucumber, peeled if not organic
1 large leaf of green kale
1–2 stalks of celery
1 lemon or lime, peeled

Cut produce to fit your juicer's feed tube. Juice ingredients and stir. Pour into a glass and drink as soon as possible. Serves 1.

Green Berry Blast

1 cucumber, peeled if not organic
4 dark green leaves such as collard, chard, or kale
1 cup blueberries (if frozen, thaw first)
1 apple (green is lower in sugar)
½ lemon, peeled if not organic

Cut produce to fit your juicer's feed tube. Juice half of the cucumber. Roll the green leaves and push through the juicer with the other half of the cucumber. Turn off the machine and pour in the berries, then place the plunger on top. Turn the machine on and push the berries through. Add the apple and lemon, and juice. Stir the juice and drink as soon as possible. Serves 2.

Green Lemonade

2 apples (green is lower in sugar)
½ lemon, peeled if not organic
1 handful of your favorite greens

Cut produce to fit your juicer's feed tube. Juice all ingredients, stir, and serve as soon as possible. Serves 1.

Peppy Parsley

1 cucumber, peeled if not organic
1 carrot, scrubbed well, tops removed, ends trimmed
1 stalk celery with leaves
1 handful parsley
1 kale leaf
1 lemon, peeled if not organic

Cut produce to fit your juicer's feed tube. Juice the cucumber, carrot, and celery. Bunch up parsley and roll in kale leaf; add to juicer and push through. Then add lemon and juice. Stir and pour into a glass. Drink as soon as possible. Serves 1.

Super Green Sprout Drink

Note: Avoid alfalfa sprouts. Alfalfa is becoming one of the top GMO crops in the nation.

1 cucumber, peeled if not organic
1 stalk celery with leaves, as desired
1 small handful sprouts such as broccoli or radish
1 large handful sunflower sprouts
1 small handful buckwheat sprouts
1 lemon, peeled if not organic

Cut produce to fit your juicer's feed tube. Juice ingredients and stir. Pour into a glass and drink as soon as possible. Serves 1.

Green Recharger

1 cucumber, peeled if not organic
1 handful sunflower sprouts
1 handful buckwheat sprouts
1 small handful clover sprouts
1 kale leaf
1 large handful spinach
1 lime, peeled if not organic

Cut the cucumber to fit your juicer's feed tube. Juice half of the cucumber first. Bunch up the sprouts and wrap in the kale leaf. Turn off the machine and add them. Turn the machine back on and tap with the rest of the cucumber to gently push the sprouts and kale through, followed by spinach. Then juice the remaining cucumber and lime. Stir ingredients, pour into a glass, and drink as soon as possible. Serves 1–2.

Green Delight

2 Swiss chard leaves
1 celery stalk
1 handful spinach
1 handful parsley
1 apple (green is lower in sugar)
½ lemon, peeled if not organic

Cut produce to fit your juicer's feed tube. Roll the chard leaves and push through the juicer with the celery stalk. Add the spinach and parsley and push through juicer with the apple and lemon. Stir the juice and drink as soon as possible. Serves 1.

Wild Green Energy Cocktail

1 cucumber, peeled if not organic
1 celery stalk
1 handful wild greens such as dandelion, nettles, plantain, lamb's quarters, or sorrel
1 apple (green is lower in sugar)
1 lemon, peeled if not organic

Cut all ingredients to fit your juicer's feed tube, then juice. Stir the juice and drink as soon as possible. Serves 1.

---

3 K-Green Cocktail

2–3 kohlrabi leaves
1 kale leaf
1 kiwi fruit
1 celery stalk
1 apple (green has less sugar)
½ lemon, peeled if not organic

Cut produce to fit your juicer's feed tube. Roll the leaves and push through the juicer with the kiwi fruit and celery stalk. Add the apple and lemon, then juice. Stir the juice and drink as soon as possible. Serves 1.

Greens of Life

2 chard leaves
2 collard leaves
1 handful parsley

1 cucumber, peeled if not organic
1 lemon, peeled if not organic

Roll leaves, place parsley inside one leaf, and push through juicer with cucumber, followed by the lemon. Stir the juice and drink as soon as possible. Serves 1–2.

Goin' Green

Several beet leaves
Several kohlrabi leaves
2 stalks celery
1 cucumber, peeled if not organic
3 carrots
1 pear
½ lemon, peeled if not organic

Place some green leaves in your juicer; alternate leaves with celery followed by cucumber, carrot, pear, and lemon. Stir the juice and drink as soon as possible. Serves 1–2.

Arugula Cocktail

1 cucumber, peeled if not organic
1 handful arugula
2 stalks celery
1-inch-chunk ginger root
1 lemon, peeled if not organic

Cut cucumber in half. Juice one-half cucumber. Bunch up arugula and push through juicer with other half of the cucumber, followed by celery, ginger root, and lemon. Stir the juice and drink as soon as possible. Serves 1.

Mustard Surprise

3 carrots, scrubbed well, tops removed, ends trimmed
2 stalks celery
2–3 mustard leaves
1 cucumber, peeled if not organic
1 apple (green is lower in sugar)

Juice carrots and celery, roll mustard leaves and place in juicer. Push the greens through with the cucumber and apple. Stir the juice and drink as soon as possible. Serves 1–2.

Wheatgrass Light

1 green apple, washed
1 handful wheatgrass, rinsed
½ lemon, washed, or peeled if not organic
2–3 sprigs mint, rinsed (optional)

Cut produce to fit your juicer's feed tube. Starting with apple, juice all ingredients and stir. Pour into a glass and drink as soon as possible. Serves 1.

Wheatgrass With Coconut Water

1–2 oz. wheatgrass juice
8 oz. coconut water

Pour wheatgrass juice into a glass. Add coconut water and stir. Serves 1.

Liver-Cleansing Cocktail

3 carrots, scrubbed well, tops removed, ends trimmed
1 cucumber, peeled if not organic
1 beet with stem and leaves, scrubbed well

2 stalks celery
1 handful parsley
1- to 2-inch-chunk ginger root, scrubbed or peeled
1 lemon, peeled if not organic

Cut produce to fit your juicer's feed tube. Juice all ingredients and stir. Pour into a glass and drink as soon as possible. Serves 1–2.

WEIGHT-LOSS RECIPES

Cranberry-Pear Fat Buster

2 pears, Bartlett or Asian
½ cucumber, peeled if not organic
¼ lemon, peeled if not organic
2 tablespoons cranberries, fresh or thawed if frozen
½- to 1-inch-chunk ginger root

Cut produce to fit your juicer's feed tube. Juice ingredients and stir. Pour into a glass and drink as soon as possible. Serves 1.

NOTE: To make this a smoothie, add about 6 ice cubes and blend until creamy.

Weight-Loss Buddy

3–4 carrots, scrubbed well, tops removed, ends trimmed
1 Jerusalem artichoke, scrubbed well
1 cucumber, peeled if not organic
1 lemon, peeled if not organic
½ small beet, scrubbed well, with stems and leaves

Cut produce to fit your juicer's feed tube. Juice ingredients and stir. Pour into a glass and drink as soon as possible. Serves 1–2.

Energizing Cocktails

All the juice recipes in this book could be considered energizing, so don't feel that you are limited to this section if you want to increase your energy. I created this section to draw your attention to the fact that fresh, raw juices can greatly improve your energy. They will all help you increase the nutrients and biophotons that energize your body.

The Morning Energizer

4 carrots, scrubbed well, tops removed, ends trimmed
1 handful parsley
1 lemon, peeled if not organic
1 apple (green has less sugar)
2-inch-chunk fresh ginger root, peeled

Cut produce to fit your juicer's feed tube. Juice ingredients and stir. Pour into a glass and drink as soon as possible. Serves 1.

Energize-Your-Day Cocktail

1 apple (green is lower in sugar)
2 dark green leaves (chard, collard, or kale)
1 stalk celery with leaves
1 lemon, peeled if not organic
½ cucumber, peeled if not organic
½- to 1-inch-chunk fresh ginger root, peeled

Cut the apple into sections that fit your juicer's feed tube. Roll the green leaves and push through the feed tube with the apple, celery, lemon, cucumber, and ginger. Stir the juice and pour into a glass. Drink as soon as possible. Serves 1.

Mood Mender

Fennel juice has been used as a traditional tonic to help the body release endorphins, the "feel-good" peptides, from the brain into the bloodstream. Endorphins help to diminish anxiety and fear and generate a mood of euphoria.

3 fennel stalks with leaves
3 carrots, scrubbed well, tops removed, ends trimmed
2 stalks celery with leaves, as desired
½ pear
1-inch-chunk ginger root, peeled

Cut produce to fit your juicer's feed tube. Juice ingredients and stir. Pour into a glass and drink as soon as possible. Serves 1–2.

Happy Mood Morning

½ apple (green is lower in sugar)
4–5 carrots, well scrubbed, tops removed, ends trimmed
3 fennel stalks with leaves and flowers
½ cucumber, peeled if not organic
1 handful spinach
1-inch-chunk ginger root

Cut produce to fit your juicer's feed tube. Juice apple first and follow with other ingredients. Stir and pour into a glass; drink as soon as possible. Serves 1–2.

Smoothies

Berry Blast Smoothie

1 cucumber, peeled if not organic

½ apple

1 cup berries (blueberries, raspberries, or blackberries), fresh or frozen (thawed)

3–4 dark green leaves (collards, Swiss chard, or kale)

1-inch-chunk ginger root

½ lemon, peeled if not organic (Meyers lemons are sweeter)

1 avocado

Cut the cucumber and apple in chunks. Place the cucumber, apple, and berries in a blender and process until smooth. Chop the greens and ginger and add to the blender along with the juice of half a lemon; process until smooth. Add the avocado and process until well blended. Serves 2.

Green Coconut Delight (Yeast-Fat Buster Smoothie)

1 cucumber cut in chunks, peeled if not organic

1 cup raw spinach, kale, or chard, chopped

1 avocado, peeled, seeded, and cut in quarters

½ cup coconut milk

1 Tbsp. coconut oil

Juice of 1 lime or lemon

Combine all ingredients in a blender and process until creamy. Serves 2.

Kale-Pear Smoothie

1 cucumber, peeled if not organic

1 cup kale

2 pears (Asian or Bartlett)

1 avocado

6 ice cubes

Chop cucumber, kale, and pears and place in the blender; process until smooth. Add the avocado and ice and blend until creamy. Serves 2.

Healthy Green Smoothie

1 cucumber, peeled if not organic

2 stalks celery

1 handful kale, parsley, or spinach

1 green apple

½ lemon, peeled if not organic

6 ice cubes

Chop the cucumber, celery, greens, and apple. Place in blender with lemon and ice; process until creamy. Serves 2.

Sprouted Almond-Vanilla Smoothie

1 cup raw almonds, soaked overnight

1 cup unsweetened almond milk

1 cup berries

½ tsp. vanilla

6 ice cubes

Soak almonds in water overnight so that they will sprout. (Sprouting allows the almond to partially germinate, which removes the enzyme inhibitors and increases nutrient value.) Blend together almonds, almond milk, berries, vanilla, and ice. Pour in glasses and serve as soon as possible. Serves 2.

Nutty Delight

10 raw almonds
1 Tbsp. sunflower seeds
1 Tbsp. sesame seeds
1 Tbsp. flaxseed
1 Tbsp. chia seeds (optional)
1 cup pineapple juice (juice half a pineapple)
1 cup chopped parsley
½ cup milk of choice
½ tsp. pure vanilla extract
1 Tbsp. protein powder (optional)
6 ice cubes

Place the nuts, seeds, and pineapple juice in a bowl; cover and soak overnight. Place this nut and seed mixture with the juice in a blender and add the parsley, milk, vanilla, protein powder (as desired), and ice cubes. Blend on high speed until smooth. This drink will be a bit chewy because of the nuts and seeds. Serves 2.

Dr. Nina's Sweet Dandelion Smoothie

1 pear, Bartlett or Asian
1 apple (green has less sugar)
1 large handful dandelion greens
1 cup coconut milk
Juice of ½ lemon
¼ cup flaxseeds
6 ice cubes (optional)

Place all ingredients in a blender and process until a creamy shake. Serves 2.

Soups

Quick Energy Soup

1 cup fresh carrot juice (5–7 medium carrots, or
     approximately 1 pound, yield about 1 cup)
1 lemon, peeled
1-inch-chunk ginger root
1 avocado, peeled and seed removed
½ tsp. ground cumin

Juice the carrots, lemon, and ginger. Pour the juice in a blender. Add the avocado and cumin and blend until smooth. Serve chilled. Serves 1.

Cherie's Yummy Energy Soup

2–3 carrots, scrubbed
2–3 stalks celery with leaves, as desired
½ cucumber, peeled if not organic
½ lemon, peeled
1 handful parsley
1–2-inch-chunk ginger root, peeled
1 avocado, peeled and seeded
Garnish options: grated zucchini, chopped fresh corn,
     or crunchy sprouts such as pea, lentil, and bean

Juice the carrots, celery, cucumber, lemon, parsley, and ginger root. Pour the juice in a blender and add the avocado. Blend until smooth. Pour into bowls and serve immediately. You may garnish with any of the optional additions for a crunchy topper. Serves 2.

Skinny Shake

1 cucumber, peeled and cut in chunks
1 stalk celery, juiced or chopped into small pieces
Juice of 1 lemon
½ tsp. freshly grated lemon peel

Place the cucumber chunks in a freezer bag and freeze them until solid. Combine the cucumber chunks in a blender with the celery, lemon juice, and lemon peel. Blend on high speed until smooth. Serves 1.

Borscht in the Raw

6 tomatoes
2 beets
3 carrots
3 stalks celery
2 Tbsp. lemon juice
3 oranges, peeled, or 1 peach
1 Tbsp. raw honey or 4 dates, pitted
½ cup extra-virgin olive oil
½ cup chopped parsley
1–2 cups water, as needed
1 cup raw walnuts
½ head cabbage and 1 beet, grated and set aside for later

Juice the tomatoes, beets, carrots, and celery together. In a blender, combine the juice plus lemon juice, peeled oranges or peach, sweetener, olive oil, parsley, and water, if needed. Pulse in the walnuts, leaving a nutty consistency. Pour in individual serving dishes and add the grated cabbage and beets into each one. Serves 2.

Red Bell Pepper Soup

¼ cup water
Juice of ½ lemon
1 small cucumber, peeled if not organic
1 green onion, chopped
⅓ cup parsley, chopped
⅓ cup cilantro, chopped
1 clove garlic
2 Tbsp. extra-virgin olive oil
1 pinch Celtic sea salt
1 large red bell pepper

Blend all ingredients together in a blender until smooth. Serves 2.

Icy Spicy Gazpacho

2 tomatoes, cut in chunks
1 cup fresh carrot juice (about 5–7 carrots)
1 lemon, juiced, peeled if putting it through a juice machine
½ bunch cilantro, rinsed and chopped
¼ teaspoon Celtic sea salt
¼ teaspoon ground cumin
¼ small jalapeño, chopped (more if you like it hot)

Place the tomato chunks in a freezer bag and freeze until solid. Pour the carrot and lemon juices into a blender and add the frozen tomato chunks, cilantro, salt, cumin, and jalapeño. Blend on high speed until smooth, but slushy; serve immediately. Serves 2.

Vegetable Medley

2 cups water or vegetable broth
1 cup green beans, chopped
1 cup asparagus, chopped
2 carrots, chopped
2 stalks celery, chopped
½ onion, chopped
1 tsp. Celtic sea salt
Pinch of mace (optional)

Pour water or vegetable broth into a soup pot. Add the vegetables and gently warm for about 10 minutes, or until vegetables are just slightly tender. Pour into a blender, add the mace, if using, and sea salt, and blend well. Pour into bowls. Serves 2.

Creamy Red Pepper Soup

3 large red bell peppers
6 garlic cloves
1 cup almond, oat, or rice milk
1 Tbsp. balsamic vinegar
2 tsp. Celtic sea salt
6 fresh basil leaves, rinsed
Garnish: chopped fresh basil (optional)

Lightly steam the peppers and garlic for about 5 minutes or just until tender. Cut the peppers into chunks. Pour the milk into a blender and add the peppers, garlic, balsamic vinegar, salt, and basil. Blend on high speed until smooth. Pour into bowls and garnish with fresh basil, as desired. Serve immediately. Serves 1–2.

Beyond the Weekend Breakfasts

Buckwheat Granola

½ cup fresh orange juice

¼ cup raw honey or pure maple syrup, adjust to taste

2 tsp. vanilla

1 tsp. cinnamon

1 apple, chopped (optional)

1 cup dried coconut

1 cup chopped raw almonds

1 cup chopped raw walnuts

1 cup raw sunflower seeds

1 cup raw sesame seeds

1 cup wheat germ

2 cups Sprouted Buckwheat Groats (see recipe)

Mix orange juice, honey, vanilla, cinnamon, and apple (if using) in blender. Set aside.

In a bowl, place coconut, almonds, walnuts, sunflower seeds, sesame seeds, wheat germ, and dehydrated buckwheat groats. Pour the blended ingredients over the entire mixture and toss well to coat all the dry ingredients.

Scoop in clumps onto ParaFlexx sheets. Dehydrate at 105 degrees for about 8 hours or until tops are crunchy. Turn over and dehydrate until tops are crunchy. Makes 6 cups.

Apple Muesli

½ cup raisins

¼ cup rolled oats

2 Tbsp. sunflower seeds

2 Tbsp. flaxseed

2 Tbsp. bee pollen

½ tsp. ascorbic acid (vitamin C powder)

½ cup milk of choice

½ cup chopped apple

½ tsp. cinnamon extract or ground cinnamon

Place raisins, oats, sunflower seeds, flaxseed, bee pollen, and ascorbic acid in a bowl and cover with milk. Cover the bowl and let soak overnight in the refrigerator. Add chopped apple and cinnamon before serving. Makes about 1½ cups.

Lemon Muesli

¼ cup rolled oats

¼ cup raisins

2 Tbsp. almonds

2 Tbsp. flaxseed

½ teaspoon ascorbic acid (vitamin C powder)

½ cup milk of choice

1 Tbsp. fresh lemon juice

1 tsp. freshly grated lemon peel, preferably organic

Place the oats, raisins, almonds, flaxseed, and vitamin C in a bowl; pour the milk over them. Cover the bowl and refrigerate overnight. Add the lemon juice and zest and stir before serving. Makes about 1 cup.

Sprouted Buckwheat Groats

Put 1 cup (or as much as you want) of raw buckwheat groat seeds into a bowl or your sprouter. Add 2–3 times as much cool, purified water. Swish seeds around to assure even water contact for all. Allow seeds to soak for 1 to 2 hours. Note: Groats take up all the water they need quickly, which is why their soak time is short. Don't over-soak since they get waterlogged if soaked too long and won't sprout. Drain off the soak water. Rinse thoroughly with cool water. Groats create very starchy water; it's very thick! They won't sprout well unless rinsed well, so rinse until the water runs clear. Drain thoroughly. You can add to your sprouter at this time or simply put the sprouts in a colander and cover with a tea towel. Set out of direct sunlight at room temperature (70 degrees is optimal). Rinse and drain again in 4–8 hours. Yields approximately 1½ cups of sprouts.

For your morning cereal, sprouted buckwheat is great served with rice, oat, or almond milk and a sprinkle of ground almonds and cinnamon.

Guilt-Free "Bacon"

¼ cup extra-virgin olive oil
4 Tbsp. apple cider vinegar
2 Tbsp. raw honey
1 tsp. ground black pepper
1 eggplant, thinly sliced into strips

Mix together the olive oil, vinegar, honey, and pepper, and marinate the eggplant strips for at least 2 hours in the mixture. Then place the strips on a dehydrator sheet and dehydrate for 12 hours at 105–115 degrees. Turn strips over and dehydrate another 12 hours.

Salads

Walnut Zucchini Greens

1 head of broccoli (lightly blanch broccoli florets
    under hot tap water until they turn bright green)
2 small zucchini, finely shredded in food processor
1 red pepper, finely chopped
2 cups torn romaine or green leaf lettuce
½ cup walnuts, chopped
Ginger-Lime Dressing (see recipe)

Mix first three ingredients in bowl. Then place
veggies on the bed of greens. Sprinkle walnuts over
top. Drizzle dressing over salad. Serves 4.

Apple Fennel Salad With Lemon Zest

2 cups fennel, sliced julienne thin
2 cups apple, sliced julienne thin
2 Tbsp. fresh lemon juice
2 Tbsp. lemon zest
2 Tbsp. extra-virgin olive oil
2 Tbsp. fresh, minced thyme
1 sliver of jalapeño, minced
1 tsp. Celtic sea salt

Place the fennel and apple slices in a bowl; set aside.
In a small bowl, whisk together lemon juice, zest,
olive oil, thyme, jalapeño, and salt. Pour dressing
over fennel-apple mixture and toss. Serves 4.

Winter Salad

1 large grapefruit
2 small fresh fennel bulbs, trimmed, halved vertically,

sliced paper-thin (save discarded parts for juicing)
1 cup fresh parsley, chopped
Lemon-Ginger Dressing (see recipe)

Peel grapefruit and cut off white part. Separate segments and slice in pieces. Combine grapefruit, fennel, and parsley. Add dressing to taste and toss. Serves 2.

Dr. Nina's Russian Cabbage Slaw

4 cups shredded cabbage
1 cup grated carrot
½ cup dandelion greens or watercress, chopped
4 cloves garlic, minced
Juice of ½ lemon
¼ cup extra-virgin olive oil

Place the cabbage, carrot, greens, and garlic in a bowl; set aside. In a small bowl, whisk together lemon juice and olive oil. Pour over the cabbage mixture and toss well. Serves 4.

Sprouted Quinoa Salad

2 cups sprouted quinoa
2 avocados, diced
2 tomatoes, diced
1 clove garlic minced
½ cup chopped cilantro (optional)
3 Tbsp. nutritional yeast
1 tsp. cumin
½ tsp. Celtic sea salt
Juice of 1 lime

Soak quinoa overnight and then sprout for 2 days.

Put quinoa in a bowl with remaining ingredients. Toss and serve on a bed of greens or in raw burritos. Serves 4.

Broccoli-Cauliflower Slaw

1 cup broccoli florets
1 cup cauliflower florets
½ red sweet onion, chopped
1 carrot, chopped
½ tsp. Celtic sea salt
Pinch of dill weed
½ cup Cashew Mayonnaise (see recipe)

Put all ingredients except mayonnaise in the food processor and pulse until they are like "slaw." Stir in Cashew Mayonnaise. Serves 2.

DRESSINGS, SAUCES, DIPS, AND CONDIMENTS

Sesame Dressing

½ cup sesame oil
1 Tbsp. grated ginger
1 Tbsp. tamari
4 cloves minced garlic
¼ cup rice vinegar
1 Tbsp. pure maple syrup
1 tsp. mustard
Dash of cayenne pepper
¼–½ cup purified water, as desired

Place all ingredients in a blender and process until smooth. Makes about 1¼ cups.

Sunflower Dill Sauce

2 cups raw sunflower seeds, soaked for 8–12 hours
⅔ cup lemon juice or 1 cucumber, peeled
⅓ cup extra-virgin olive oil
2 Tbsp. minced garlic
1 tsp. Celtic sea salt
6 Tbsp. fresh, chopped dill or 2 Tbsp. dried dill

In a high-speed blender, blend sunflower seeds, lemon juice or cucumber, olive oil, garlic, and salt until smooth. Pulse in the dill. More cucumber may be added for desired consistency if needed. Makes about 3 cups.

Ginger-Lime Dressing

¼ cup fresh lime juice
¼ cup sesame oil
¼ cup purified water
2 Tbsp. tamari
2 Tbsp. fresh mint
1 Tbsp. fresh cilantro
1 tsp. ginger root
1 thin slice red chili pepper or dash of cayenne pepper
1 Tbsp. pure maple syrup
1 tsp. Celtic sea salt

Combine all the ingredients in a blender and blend well. Makes about 1 cup.

Lemon-Ginger Dressing

2 lemons, juiced
2-inch-chunk ginger root, grated

½ cup extra-virgin olive oil

2 cloves garlic, peeled and crushed

3 Tbsp. miso

2 Tbsp. shoyu

2–3 Tbsp. raw honey or pure maple syrup

Mix all ingredients in blender. If needed, add water to thin. Makes 1 cup.

Cashew Mayonnaise

1 cup raw cashews, soaked overnight

Juice of 1 lemon

1 tsp. Celtic sea salt

½ tsp. onion powder

½ tsp. dill weed

Water as needed

Put all ingredients in blender with water just barely covering the cashews. Blend until smooth. Taste and adjust seasoning if necessary. Makes about 1½ cups.

Raw Almond Mayo

2 cups raw almonds, soaked overnight

4 Tbsp. pure maple syrup or agave syrup (also called agave nectar)

½ cup water

Juice of 2 lemons

1 teaspoon onion or garlic powder

1 tsp. Celtic sea salt

¼ cup fresh basil

¼ cup extra-virgin olive oil (optional)

In a food processor, thoroughly blend almonds with maple syrup, water, and lemon juice. Add remaining ingredients. If mixture needs to be thickened, slowly add oil while processing. Makes about 8 servings.

Mexican Almond Dip

1 cup almonds, soaked
½–1 tsp. Celtic sea salt
½ small sweet onion
½ clove elephant garlic with the center removed
¼ tsp. chili powder
¼–½ tsp. cumin
Water, as needed for desired consistency

Soak the almonds, covered, a day ahead, changing the water once. Mix all ingredients in a food processor. Serve on romaine leaves with Chef Avi Dalene's Green Tortillas (see recipe) or Awesome Corn Crackers (see recipe). Makes about 1¼ cups.

Healthy Raw Ketchup

Studies involving the tomato have cropped up all over the world. It's rich in lycopene, an antioxidant that helps fight against cancer cell formation as well as other kinds of health complications and diseases.

1 cup chopped tomato
1 cup sun-dried tomatoes, soaked for 30 minutes, drained, and chopped
1 Tbsp. fresh garlic, minced
10 fresh basil leaves
3 dates, pitted
¼ cup extra-virgin olive oil
1 Tbsp. shoyu or 1 tsp. Celtic sea salt
1–2 Tbsp. Bragg's raw, unfiltered apple cider vinegar

Blend all ingredients together until it forms a paste. Makes about 2½ cups.

Raw Pesto Sauce

½–¾ cup organic raw pine nuts
¼ cup fresh organic basil, de-stemmed
2 Tbsp. extra-virgin olive oil
1–2 Tbsp. fresh lemon juice
1–2 garlic cloves
1 tsp. Celtic sea salt
¼ cup purified water, reserved

Add all the ingredients to a food processor or blender. Pulse the mixture in food processor or blender, adding 1 tablespoon of water at a time to help facilitate blending and in order to reach the desired consistency for the sauce. Makes about 1¼ cups.

Nutty Cheese Sauce

1 cup macadamia nuts and 1 cup raw pine nuts, soaked, or 2 cups cashews, soaked (cashews are a bit sweeter and usually less expensive)
½ cup fresh lemon juice
1½ tsp. Celtic sea salt
1 Tbsp. garlic, chopped
½ tsp. ground peppercorns (optional)
Purified water as needed (usually between ¼ and ½ cup)

Soak nuts first for several hours. Blend all ingredients until very creamy. Blend for about 3 to 4 minutes for the creamiest sauce. Add water as needed. This sauce will keep 3 days in the refrigerator in a covered container. Makes 1½ cups.

Marinara Sauce

1 cup sun-dried tomatoes
1½ cups blended tomatoes
2 Tbsp. chopped onion
2 cloves garlic, peeled
2 Tbsp. extra-virgin olive oil
½ cup fresh lemon juice
Celtic sea salt, to taste

Combine all the ingredients in a blender and process until desired consistency is reached. Makes about 3 cups.

Almond Filling

2 cups almonds, soaked 7–8 hours, rinsed well
1 carrot, with cut ends and peeled, chopped (if using food processor)
2 stalks celery, cut ends, finely minced
1 medium red pepper, finely minced, with seeds and ribs removed
1 small onion, finely minced

Using a juicer with a blank blade such as the Champion or the Omega, or a food processor, homogenize the almonds and carrot, catching them in a large bowl. Or place the soaked almonds and carrot in a food processor and blend until homogenized. To this mixture add celery, red pepper, and onion. Thoroughly knead, integrating all ingredients with your hands. Makes about 3 cups.

DEHYDRATED FOODS

Dehydrated foods make great snacks for work, travel, and kids' lunches. They help you lose weight much more easily because they offer taste satisfaction without a lot of calories. It doesn't take much time to prepare them, and the rewards are great.

You'll notice that the dehydration temperature is 105 degrees for almost all dehydrated foods, which preserves nutrients, vitamins, and enzymes. There are a number of schools of thought as to what the best temperature is (between 105 and 118 degrees) to preserve the most enzymes and vitamins. When in doubt, choose the lower temperature setting on your dehydrator. (If you need a dehydrator, see Appendix A.)

Spicy Kale Chips

1 bunch curly kale
¼ cup apple cider or coconut vinegar
¼ cup fresh lemon juice
¼ cup extra-virgin olive oil
Pinch of cayenne pepper or red pepper flakes
2 tsp. garlic, minced or pressed
½ tsp. Celtic sea salt

Wash the kale and then cut it into 3-inch-long strips and set aside to dry.

Add vinegar, lemon juice, olive oil, and cayenne pepper or red pepper flakes to a blender and process on high speed until well combined. Pour the marinade into a bowl. Then dip the kale leaves in the marinade one at a time and massage the marinade into the leaf. Shake off excess marinade and place kale pieces on dehydrator ParaFlexx sheets. Sprinkle with garlic and sea salt, and dehydrate for 4 to 8 hours at 105 degrees or until crisp. (Chips will get smaller as they dry.) Makes about 4 trays of chips.

Flax Crackers

2 cups flaxseeds
1 red bell pepper
1 carrot
½ cup sun-dried tomatoes
2 cups fresh tomatoes
Juice of 1 lemon
1 clove fresh garlic
1 Tbsp. shoyu or Bragg's liquid aminos or 1–2 tsp. Celtic sea salt

Blend all ingredients together in a food processor. Add water if the batter is too dry. Press mixture flat onto a ParaFlexx sheet into a large square that covers the sheet. Make sure that the mixture stands only about ⅛-inch high. The thicker the cracker, the chewier it is and the longer it takes to dry. With a knife or spatula, score the batch to the size you'd like before dehydrating. (A typical square is 3x3.) Dehydrate around 105 degrees overnight; flip over once one side is dry. Dehydrate until completely dry. Store in an airtight container. Makes about 27 crackers.

Nan's Carrot Curry Flax Krax

½–1 cup ground golden flaxseeds
1½ cups carrot juice
½–1 cup warm water
½-inch-chunk ginger root
1–2 tsp. orange zest

1 garlic clove
½ tsp. Celtic sea salt
1 Tbsp. onion, chopped
1 tsp. dried cilantro

Soak flaxseed for 2 or more hours. While seeds are soaking, juice carrots to get 1 ½ cups juice. Pour juice in a blender or food processor. Add all the other ingredients and blend until well combined. Batter should be the consistency of pancake batter. Add water as needed if it is too dry. Pour onto a ParaFlexx tray. Score into desired cracker size. Dry at 105 degrees until crisp and breaks easily into pieces. Makes approximately 12 crackers.

Nan's Zesty Green Berry Krax

1 cup green grapes
1 cup blackberries
1 cup raspberries or strawberries
¼-inch-round-slice of organic lemon with skin
½-inch-chunk ginger
1 large Granny Smith apple, chopped
2–3 Tbsp. barley green powder (your choice of
    brands)

Blend grapes in blender or food processor. Add the remaining ingredients and process until well combined. Dry soft and pliable for fruit roll-up options. Makes about 12 crackers.

Option: For super zesty, open up and sprinkle 3 teabags of Celestial Seasons Red Zinger or Berry Zinger herbal tea into the mixture.

Veggie Nut Crackers

1½ cups almonds, soaked overnight
1½ cups sunflower seeds, soaked 1–2 hours
1 cup pumpkin seeds, soaked 1–2 hours
7–8 cups veggie pulp (2 zucchini, 4 grated carrots, or
    pulp left over from juicing 4 carrots, 2 stalks celery,
    2 red bell peppers, 1 small red onion chopped)
2 small Roma tomatoes, chopped
½ cup chopped fresh basil
½ cup chopped cilantro
Juice of ½ lemon
3 tsp. veggie seasoning
½ tsp. cayenne pepper
2–3 tsp. Celtic sea salt
2 tsp. dried dill

Drain water from nuts and seeds. Place almonds in a food processor, and add sunflower and pumpkin seeds; use the S blade and process until smooth in consistency. Set aside in a bowl.

Put all the chopped or grated veggies in the food processor; add the Roma tomatoes, basil, cilantro, and lemon juice.

Put the veggie mixture in with the nuts and seed mixture and combine well. Add spices and mix well.

Spread over ParaFlexx sheets ⅓ inch thick, and score before dehydrating. Dehydrate for 16–20 hours at 105 degrees. Time will vary. Makes about 36 crackers.

Awesome Corn Crackers

½ cup golden flaxseeds, soaked 4–8 hours in 2 cups
    purified water
½ cup raw almonds, soaked, covered, 8 hours in
    purified water
2 cups fresh corn cut off the cob (about 6 ears of corn)
2 Tbsp. ground cumin
2 Tbsp. chopped sweet onion
1–2 tsp. Celtic sea salt

Blend flaxseeds and almonds in a food processor;
add the other ingredients and process until mixture
reaches consistency of pancake batter. Spoon about
1 tablespoon of batter onto the ParaFlexx sheets and
swirl with a spoon until it's a thin round layer, or
cover about 4 ParaFlexx sheets with batter spread
very thin. Dehydrate 10–20 hours, depending on
desired crispness. If you have covered the ParaFlexx
sheets, you can cut crackers to the shape desired
when dry. You can also cut in strips for salads. Makes
about 36 crackers.

Tomato Flat Bread

1 cup almonds, soaked overnight
2 cups wheat berries or oat groats, soaked overnight
1 clove garlic
1 cup ground flaxseeds
1 cup tomato purée (made from fresh tomatoes)
1 cup water

The night before, soak almonds and grain (separately).
When you are ready to make the bread, drain each.
In food processor, mix the garlic and almonds until

well ground. Place in large bowl. Put wheat or oat grouts in processor and mix until a mash is created. Do not overprocess once you reach that stage. Put in the bowl with the almonds and garlic. Add flaxseeds and stir until well combined. Add tomato purée and water; mix well. Spread over two ParaFlexx sheets about ¼ inch thick. Score to desired size. Dehydrate for 1 hour at 140 degrees. Reduce heat to 105 degrees and continue to dry for 8 more hours or until it reaches the desired dryness. Makes about 18 crackers.

MAIN COURSES

Garlic Dijon Halibut

1–1½ lb. halibut, cut into 4 pieces
¼ cup lemon juice
Celtic sea salt and pepper to taste

Topping

2 Tbsp. mayonnaise
2 Tbsp. green onions, chopped
2 tsp. fresh lemon juice
2 garlic cloves, pressed or minced
1 tsp. Dijon mustard
¼ tsp. hot sauce or pinch of cayenne pepper

On each side of the halibut, make 3 diagonal cuts 2 inches long and ½ inch deep. Place the halibut in a large shallow dish and pour the lemon juice over it. Marinate for 30 minutes at room temperature. Preheat the oven to 450 degrees. Place the fish on a broiling pan and sprinkle with lemon juice from the marinade. Bake the fish for 15 minutes, or until it is opaque in the center. While the fish is baking, combine the mayonnaise, green onions, lemon juice, garlic, mustard, and hot sauce or cayenne. Mix well. Remove fish from oven when done. Turn the oven to broil. Sprinkle fish with salt and pepper. Spread the topping over the fish and broil for 2 minutes, or until the topping is golden brown. Serves 4.

Squash and Arugula Enchiladas

Delicata squash is my favorite in this recipe. It features yellow skin with green stripes on an oblong shape. A ¾-cup portion contains just 30 calories, so it's a great choice if you want to lose weight. It's also a good source of vitamin C and carotenes. Adding arugula or watercress gives you an example of combining cooked and living food.

2 delicata squash, 1 acorn squash, or ¼ butternut
    squash (other winter squash, sweet potatoes, or
    yams can be substituted)
1 cup brown rice, cooked
1 Tbsp. virgin coconut oil
4–6 tortillas (sprouted whole grain, spelt, or gluten
    free)
½–1 cup arugula, chopped
Salt and pepper to taste

Bake the delicata squash in a preheated oven set at 400 degrees for 30 minutes or until tender but not soft. Add water about an inch deep to the baking pan, and the squash cooks faster. While the squash is baking, cook the rice. (If you want meat in this dish, you can reduce the rice to ½ cup and add ½ pound of cooked ground meat.) When the squash is tender, remove from the oven and cut in half. If you are not using delicata squash, scoop out the seeds and peel; however, if you are using delicata and the skin is tender, you don't need to peel. Cut the squash in chunks and mix with rice; add seasoning to taste and set aside; keep warm.

In a large skillet, heat the oil. Heat the tortillas one at a time until warm and slightly browned, but be careful not to overcook or they will get crisp and won't roll into an enchilada. Spoon 2–3 tablespoons of the squash-rice mixture into the center of each tortilla and spread from one end to the other. Add arugula to the top of that mixture, adding salt and pepper to taste, and roll each side toward the center. Serve hot. Serves 4–6.

Stuffed Bell Peppers

6 medium carrots, chopped
1–2 celery stalks, chopped
1 large or 2 small ripe avocados
1 tsp. dulse or Celtic sea salt
½ cup chopped cucumber
½ cup chopped tomato
½ tsp. cumin
1 large red or yellow bell pepper
Raw sunflower seeds for garnish

Place carrots and celery in a food processor and process until pulp consistency, or use carrot and celery pulp leftover from juicing. Transfer the pulp to a bowl. Remove the flesh from the avocado(s) and, using a fork, mash the avocado into the carrot-celery pulp. Add the dulse or salt, cucumber, tomato, and cumin, and mix well. Cut bell pepper in half; scoop out the seeds and stuff with the carrot-avocado mixture. Top each stuffed pepper with 1 tsp. of sunflower seeds. Serves 2.

Sunshine "Eggless" Salad or Sunshine "Eggless" Salad Roll-ups

½ cup pure water
½ cup fresh lemon juice
1½ tsp. turmeric
1 tsp. Celtic sea salt, adjust to taste
1½ cups raw macadamia nuts or cashews (sweeter with cashews)
½ cup green onion, diced
½ cup celery, diced
⅓ cup red bell pepper, diced (optional)

Place all ingredients (except diced green onion, celery, and red bell pepper) into a food processor, fitted with an S blade. Process until very smooth. Transfer to a bowl and add the green onion, celery, and red bell pepper. Mix well.

Serve as a dip with veggies or place onto romaine lettuce leaves for a quick and easy wrap. May be served as an appetizer also. Cut cucumber slices diagonally and lay out onto service platter. Place 1 Tbsp. of Sunshine "Eggless" Salad onto each cucumber slice. Garnish with sprigs of fresh parsley or sliced green onion. Serves 16–20 appetizer size; 8–10 as roll-up sandwich.

Carrot Sauce With Asparagus and Fresh Peas Over Rice

1 cup brown rice or quinoa

1½ cups carrot juice (about 8–11 carrots)

½ cup raw cashews

2 Tbsp. white or yellow miso

1 pound fresh asparagus

½ cup fresh or frozen peas

2 scallions, chopped

¼ cup marinated sun-dried tomato halves, thinly sliced

2 cloves garlic, pressed

3 Tbsp. fresh basil, finely chopped

Cook brown rice or quinoa according to directions.

While rice is cooking, combine the carrot juice, cashews, and miso in a blender or food processor, blending on high until the cashews are no longer gritty and the mixture is smooth and creamy. Snap off the tops of the asparagus. Cut the tender upper portion into 1-inch pieces. In a medium-size skillet, combine the carrot juice mixture and asparagus. Bring to a boil and then reduce the heat to simmer, stirring occasionally for 2–3 minutes. Add the peas and simmer until the asparagus is just tender, about 2 minutes. Add the scallions, sun-dried tomatoes, and garlic, mixing well; simmer for 1–2 minutes. Remove the sauce from the heat.

Divide the rice or quinoa in 4 portions. Top each portion with about ¼ of the sauce and sprinkle chopped basil on top of each portion. Serves 4.

Nicole's Stuffed Acorn Squash

1 acorn squash
½ cup grass-fed ground turkey
¼ cup quinoa
1–2 garlic cloves, pressed
1 tsp. dried basil
½–1 tsp. Celtic sea salt
½ tsp. cumin
½ tsp. paprika
Broccoli-Cauliflower Slaw (see recipe)
Red bell pepper strips

Bake the acorn squash at 400 degrees for 20 minutes. Remove from oven; cut squash in half and scoop out seeds. Return to oven and bake for 25 minutes, or until tender. Adding a little water to the baking pan will speed the baking process.

While the squash is baking, cook the ground turkey and quinoa in separate pans. When cooked, scoop the turkey and quinoa into a bowl and add the basil, salt, cumin, and paprika. Stir until well combined. Scoop half the mixture into each half of the acorn squash. Top each squash with a scoop of Broccoli-Cauliflower Slaw and several red bell pepper strips. Serves 2.

Cherie's Nut Burgers

½ cup pecans or walnuts
¼ cup sunflower seeds
¼ cup hemp seeds
½ cup chia or flaxseeds (grind well)
½ cup sun-dried tomatoes, soaked 1 hour, drained and sliced

1 Tbsp. ginger, peeled and minced

2–3 cloves fresh garlic, pressed or minced

1 tsp. Celtic sea salt

2 carrots, chopped

1 stalk celery, chopped

½ cup red or yellow pepper, stemmed, seeded, chopped

½ cup zucchini, chopped

¼–½ cup dates, pitted and chopped

¼ sweet onion, chopped

¼ cup chopped parsley

1 Tbsp. fresh lemon juice

1 Tbsp. fresh oregano or 1 tsp. dried

1 Tbsp. water

Process the nuts and sunflower seeds in a food processor until ground fine. Add the hemp seeds and grind thoroughly. Set aside in a large bowl. Add the chia or flaxseeds to the ground nut and seed mixture; stir to mix.

Process the sun-dried tomatoes, ginger, garlic, and salt in the food processor. Add the carrots, celery, bell pepper, zucchini, dates, onion, parsley, lemon juice, oregano, and water. Process until well combined, but not mushy. Transfer the vegetable mixture to the ground nut and seed mixture.

Place half the mixture back in the food processor and pulse several times to mix well. Transfer to a new bowl. Repeat with remaining mixture.

Form patties with ⅓ cup of the mixture. Dehydrate patties for 1 hour at 140 degrees. Reduce the temperature to 105 degrees and dehydrate for 4 hours or until top is dry. Flip the burgers and dehydrate another 4 hours or until as dry as desired. Serve with Healthy Raw Ketchup (see recipe) and a slice of Tomato Flat Bread (see recipe), as desired. Makes about 36 burgers.

Sunny Delight Enchiladas With Corn Tortillas

5 ears of corn with kernels cut off the cob
2 Tbsp. psyllium husk (not seed)
Purified water as needed
Nan's Sunflower Pate (see recipe)
Nutty Cheese Sauce (see recipe)

Place the corn and psyllium husk in a food processor and blend until smooth; add water as needed. Batter should be about the consistency of pancake batter. Place large spoonfuls of batter on dehydrator ParaFlexx sheets. Using a spoon, swirl batter in a circular motion to shape into rounds to your desired tortilla size. Dehydrate about 4 hours at 105 degrees. Flip tortillas and dehydrate another 2 hours or until no longer wet yet soft and easy to roll. Don't leave in the dehydrator too long, or the tortillas will get hard. If that happens, you can make tostadas. Makes 16–20 tortillas.

To assemble tortillas:

Arrange tortillas on counter or breadboard. Top each tortilla with about 1 tablespoon of Nan's Sunflower Pate. Place a tablespoon of Nutty Cheese Sauce or guacamole on top of the filling; roll each tortilla into an enchilada style roll. It can be served with salsa or guacamole, as desired.

Chef Avi Dalene's Green Tortillas

1 cup chia seeds, unsoaked

4 cups zucchini (either with skins or peeled)

1 yellow or red bell pepper (red bell pepper will produce darker tortilla color)

1 tsp. coriander

1 tsp. cumin

1 tsp. quality mineralized salt (Celtic sea or Himalayan salt)

Jalapeño pepper to taste (green jalapeño peppers are unripe) or a pinch of dried red pepper flakes

¼ cup young Thai coconut water (optional)

2 Tbsp. fresh lime juice (optional)

2 tsp. ultimate clear agave nectar (optional)

Using a high-speed blender, grind chia seeds into fine powder and set aside.

Place the zucchini, bell pepper, coriander, cumin, salt, jalapeño, and pepper into a high-speed blender and process until smooth. Add ground chia powder to mixture in high-speed blender and mix gently to dough/paste consistency.

If using, add young Thai coconut water, lime juice, and ultimate clear agave nectar (may need more or less) and mix until well combined.

Divide into 10 equal portions and spread onto ParaFlexx dehydrator sheets. Starting at one corner, add the mixture to the appropriate thickness and shape into tortillas. Make them about ¼ inch thick. Continue over the entire ParaFlexx sheets until all the batter is used.

Dehydrate at 115 degrees for about 5 hours, or until desired dryness is reached. (They should be dry but flexible and soft. Do not over-dehydrate, or they will be hard.) Let set for several hours until you are ready to use them.

When dehydrating, if the tortillas get too crisp, dampen them slightly by spritzing them with a bit of good quality water. Also, the tortillas can be placed in the dehydrator to crisp up if they become moist while in storage.

Yields about 2½ dehydrator trays and makes 10 large tortillas, 40 taquito wraps, or some combination of the two.

Gourmet Pesto Pizza With Raw Buckwheat Groat Pizza Dough

2 cups sprouted buckwheat groats
1–2 garlic cloves, chopped
¾ cup finely grated carrots (or use carrot pulp)
¾ cup soaked flaxseeds (soak overnight; they'll expand to about 1½ cups) or use ground flaxseeds and extra water
½ cup extra-virgin olive oil
1 Tbsp. Italian seasonings (or fresh herbs to taste)
1–2 tsp. Celtic sea salt
Water as needed (usually ½–1 cup)
1–1½ cups Raw Pesto Sauce (see recipe)

Mix all ingredients together in a food processor. Start with buckwheat groats and garlic, followed by the rest of the ingredients. Coat a dehydrator sheet with a small amount of olive oil and scoop batches of dough (about a heaping tablespoon each) onto dehydrator sheets, swirling each scoop with a spoon to make rounds. You can make large pizza dough (about

6 inches in diameter)—or you can make smaller individual rounds (about 3 inches in diameter). The smaller rounds are easier to serve and eat. Press out the dough evenly to about ⅛ to ¼ inch thick by patting the top with your fingertips or swirling with a spoon. If it gets too sticky, dip your fingers into some water to which you add a little olive oil. Once crust is pressed out evenly, dehydrate at 105–115 degrees for about 7 hours. Flip the crackers and dry another 7–10 hours or until crust is completely dry and crisp. (It should be crunchy for the best-tasting cracker.) To speed the drying process, transfer to the mesh rack. Use a spatula when lifting dough, and be careful when transferring it not to break the crackers. Makes 36 crackers.

Top with Raw Pesto Sauce. You can also top with Nutty Cheese Sauce (see recipe) or Marinara Sauce (see recipe).

NOTE: To sprout buckwheat, soak 1 cup raw buckwheat groats for about 2 hours; it will expand to about 2 cups. Drain and rinse well. Place on counter in a colander covered with a lightweight dishtowel or in a sprouter for one day. Rinse several times while sprouting. (If you don't have time to sprout, you can use buckwheat that has been soaked for 2 hours.)

NOTE: If crust is very dry and stored in a cool dry, airtight container, it can be kept fresh for several months.

Raw Zucchini Noodles With Marinara Sauce

6 to 8 firm zucchini and/or yellow crookneck squash
1 cup Marinara Sauce (see recipe)

Fresh basil, chopped, to taste (optional)
Avocado slices (optional)

Use a vegetable spiral slicer or spirooli to make thin, long noodles out of zucchini. If possible, make zucchini noodles about six hours before serving, and let noodles sit in a bowl, uncovered, at room temperature, which can improve their texture.

Pour Marinara Sauce over the noodles, give the noodles and sauce a good toss, and serve. Top with chopped fresh basil and/or slices of avocado. Serves 3 to 4.

You can also use Raw Pesto Sauce (see recipe). Or you can make my favorite—a simple pasta dish of zucchini noodles tossed with several tablespoons of extra-virgin olive oil, 2–3 cloves of pressed garlic, ¼ cup halved sun-dried olives, and ¼ cup chopped fresh basil. Sprinkle with salt, to taste, and serve.

Nan's Sunflower Pate

3 cups sunflower seeds, soaked 8 to 12 hours; rinse
    and sprout about 4 hours
1 cup fresh lemon juice
½ cup scallions, chopped
¼–½ cup raw tahini
¼ cup liquid aminos or shoyu
2–4 slices red onion, cut into chunks
4–6 Tbsp. parsley, chopped
2–3 medium cloves garlic
½ tsp. cayenne pepper
1–2 Tbsp. ginger, chopped
1 tsp. cumin

Blend all ingredients in food processor until all the ingredients are smooth and creamy. This mixture should be on the thick side rather than thin. Add a bit of water as needed. Makes 7–8 cups.

Mock "Salmon" Pate

2 cups walnuts
2 carrots, grated, or use carrot pulp
2 ribs celery
1 large red bell pepper
2 green onions
1 large handful fresh parsley
½–1 tsp. Celtic sea salt
Raw Almond Mayo (see recipe)
Almond slivers or slices (optional)

In a food processor, mix all ingredients together until smooth. Serve on a bed of lettuce with a dollop of Raw Almond Mayo or use as filling for stuffed tomatoes or stuffed avocados. Top with almond slivers or slices. Serves 6–8.

Marinated Collard Greens

4 Tbsp. extra-virgin olive oil
Juice of 1 to 2 lemons
1–2 cloves garlic, finely minced
1 bunch fresh collard greens, washed; remove tough stems and trim out center vein

Place extra-virgin olive oil, lemon juice, and garlic in a small bowl and whisk together. Set aside.

Place collard leaves in large rectangular dish, alternating the direction of the leaves as you overlap and stack them. Pour in olive oil mixture, coating all leaves. Set aside for 3 hours before serving. Serves 10–12.

Almond Roulade

Marinated Collard Greens (see recipe)
Almond Filling (see recipe)

Take collard greens and spread 2–3 tablespoons Almond Filling on one side of each leaf. Roll each collard leaf, forming roulade. Repeat this process, using up all Almond Filling and collard greens. Cut each roulade in half or thirds and serve one to two per person. Serves 10–12.

Almond Falafel

3 cups almonds, soaked
1½ cups sunflower seeds, soaked
Juice of 2 lemons
4 cloves garlic, finely chopped
½ cup raw tahini
1½ Tbsp. curry
3 cups of greens such as parsley, cilantro, or kale, finely chopped (use food processor or finely mince)

Soak nuts and seeds for several hours. Put drained, soaked almonds in food processor and chop fine. Set aside in a medium bowl. Process the soaked sunflower seeds and put in the bowl, adding lemon juice. Add garlic, tahini, curry, and greens. Mix everything together and massage with hands. Shape into small patties and serve fresh, or dehydrate at

105 degrees for 4–5 hours. Serve with the Sunflower
Dill Sauce (see recipe). Makes 6 servings.

Zucchini Hummus

2 medium zucchini

2 tsp. olive oil

4 garlic cloves, 1 tsp. Celtic sea salt, or 1 tsp. dulse
    flakes

½ cup lemon or lime juice

½ cup sesame seeds

½ cup tahini

⅛ tsp. cayenne

1 tsp. paprika

1 tsp. cumin

Blend zucchini, oil, and garlic in food processor.
Add remaining ingredients and blend. Serves 10–12.

Mango Salsa

3 cups tomatoes, diced

3 cups fresh mango, diced

½ cup onion, minced

½ cup cilantro, chopped

2 limes, juiced

1 garlic clove, minced

1 tsp. jalapeño, minced

½ tsp. Celtic sea salt

Mix all ingredients in a bowl and let the flavors
mingle for at least 1 hour before serving. Serves 10.

Appendix A

The Weekend Weight-Loss Resource Guide

S IGN UP FOR Cherie Calboms's free Juice Newsletter at www.juiceladyinfo.com.

Cherie's websites

- www.juiceladyinfo.com—information on juicing and weight loss
- www.cheriecalbom.com—information about Cherie's websites
- www.sleepawaythepounds.com—information about the Sleep Away the Pounds program and products
- www.gococonuts.com—information about the Coconut Diet and coconut oil

Other books by Cherie and John Calbom

These books can be ordered at any of the websites above or by calling 866-8GETWEL (866-843-8935).

- Cherie Calbom, *The Juice Lady's Turbo Diet* (Siloam)
- Cherie Calbom, *The Juice Lady's Guide to Juicing for Health* (Avery)

- Cherie Calbom with John Calbom, *Juicing, Fasting, and Detoxing for Life* (Wellness Central)
- Cherie Calbom and John Calbom, *Sleep Away the Pounds* (Wellness Central)
- Cherie Calbom, *The Wrinkle Cleanse* (Avery)
- Cherie Calbom and John Calbom, *The Coconut Diet* (Wellness Central)
- Cherie Calbom, John Calbom, and Michael Mahaffey, *The Complete Cancer Cleanse* (Thomas Nelson)
- Cherie Calbom, *The Ultimate Smoothie Book* (Wellness Central)

Juicers

Find out the best juicers recommended by Cherie Calbom. Call 866-8GETWEL (866-843-8935) or visit www.juiceladyinfo.com.

Dehydrators

Find out the best dehydrators recommended by Cherie Calbom. Call 866-8GETWEL (866-843-8935) or visit www.juiceladyinfo.com.

Lymphasizer

To view the Swing Machine (lymphasizer), visit www .juiceladyinfo.com or call 866-8GETWEL (866-843-8935).

Veggie powders

To purchase or get information on Barley Max, Carrot Juice Max, and Beet Max powders, call 866-8GETWEL (866-843-8935). (These powders are ideal for when you travel or when you can't get juice.)

Virgin coconut oil

For more information on virgin coconut oil, go to www .gococonuts.com or call 866-8GETWEL (866-843-8935). To save money, order larger sizes such as gallons or quarts, which you won't typically find in the stores.

Supplements

- Multivitamins by Thorne Research: call 866-843-8935.

- Digestive enzymes Ness Formula #4 and #16 are excellent to aid digestion. Taken between meals, they help clean up undigested proteins. With the addition of enzymes, you should notice that your hair and nails grow better. Call 866-8GETWEL (866-843-8935).

- Calcium Citrate or Calcium Citramate (contains both calcium citrate-malate and malic acid; offers good solubility and superb absorption when compared to other forms of calcium) by Thorne Research: call 866-843-8935.

- Magnesium Citrate or Magnesium Citramate (as Magnesium Citrate-Malate and malic acid) by Thorne Research: call 866-843-8935.

- Vitamin C with bioflavonoids or Buffered C Powder (contains ascorbic acid, calcium, magnesium, and potassium) by Thorne Research or Allergy Research: call 866-843-8935.

- Vitamin D_3 (1,000 or 5,000 mg) by Thorne Research: call 866-843-8935.

Colon cleanse products

Call 866-843-8935 for more information on Cherie's fiber recommendations below.

- Medibulk by Thorne (psyllium powder, prune powder, apple pectin)

- Blessed Herbs Colon Cleanse Kit: After years of eating standard food, it's quite common to build up a layer of mucoid plaque—hardened mucus-like material and food residue that can coat the gastrointestinal tract. Nutrients are absorbed through the intestinal wall. The plaque hinders our ability to absorb nutrients, which can lead to numerous health problems. This colon cleanse kit contains products that can pull the plaque from your intestinal wall and carry it out of your system—Digestive Stimulator, Toxin Absorber, glass shaker jar, and user guide and dosage calendar. Specify ginger or peppermint flavor. Cost: $89.50 less 5 percent discount.

Internal cleansing kit

Blessed Herbs complete and comprehensive internal cleansing kit contains 18 items for a 21-day cleanse program with free colon cleanse kit. You get a free colon cleanse kit, along with Liver-Gallbladder Rejuvenator, Friendly Bacteria Replenisher, Parasite Cleanser, Lung Rejuvenator, Kidney and Bladder Rejuvenator, Blood and Skin Rejuvenator, and Lymph Rejuvenator, along with glass shaker jar and user guide and dosage calendar. Specify ginger or peppermint flavor. Cost $279, less 5 percent discount.

You may order Blessed Herbs cleansing products and get the 5 percent discount by calling 866-843-8935. If you want to read more about Blessed Herbs cleansing kits, go to my website www .juiceladyinfo.com. You will need to order via the toll-free number to get the discount, however.

Liver/gallbladder cleanse products

- S.A.T. by Thorne (milk thistle, artichoke, turmeric) along with Cysteplus (N-Acetyl-L-Cysteine) and Lipotropein (vitamins, minerals, L-Methionine, and herbs including dandelion, beet leaf, and black radish root)—call 866-843-8935

- Chinese herbal tinctures (4-part kit) to use with Cherie's Liver Detox Program—call 866-843-8935

Candida albicans cleanse products

- Friendly Bacteria Replenisher—visit www.juiceladyinfo .com
- Blessed Herbs Total Body Cleanse—visit www .juiceladyinfo.com or call 866-843-8935

Parasite cleanse products

- Large Para Cleanser 1 and 2 and Small Para Cleanser— visit www.juiceladyinfo.com
- Blessed Herbs Total Body Cleanse—visit www .juiceladyinfo.com or call 866-843-8935

Kidney cleanse herbs

- Blessed Herbs Kidney & Bladder Rejuvenator—call 866-843-8935

Heavy metal and toxic compounds cleanse products

For all these products, call 866-843-8935.

- Captomer by Thorne (Succinic acid from 100 mg DMSA)—chelates heavy metals
- Heavy Metal Support by Thorne—replaces important minerals and other nutrients lost during metal chelating
- Toxic Relief Booster by Thorne—nutrients designed to aid in metabolizing the increased amount of fat stored toxins released into the bloodstream during a cleanse

- Formaldehyde Relief by Thorne—provides nutrients necessary for detoxification of formaldehyde from new carpet and furniture outgassing, as well as compounds produced by *Candida albicans* or by alcohol metabolism

- Solvent Remover by Thorne—contains amino acids specific to solvent detoxification in the liver, as well as nutrients that help protect nerves from solvent damage

- Pesticide Protector by Thorne—aids in detoxification of chlorinated pesticides, organophosphates, carbamates, and pyrethrins

INFORMATION AND PRODUCTS FOR SPECIFIC DISORDERS

Sleep disorders

Testing neurotransmitters is the best way to determine if you have depletion in brain chemicals that could be causing sleep problems. Testing can be completed whether you are taking medications or not. You can determine if your neurotransmitters are out of balance by taking the Brain Wellness Programs Self Test. Just go to www.neurogistics.com and click "Get Started." Use the practitioner code SLEEP (all caps). You can order the program, which includes a urine in-home test that will yield a report on your neurotransmitter levels. You'll be given a customized protocol with guidelines for the right amino acids for you to take to help correct your imbalances. Or you can call 866-843-8935 for more information.

Beyond the Weekend: Healthy Foods List and Serving Guideline

VEGETABLES AND LEGUMES		
Choose *Prepare raw, lightly steamed, or grilled*	Limit *until you reach your weight-loss goal*	Avoid
Artichokes	Acorn squash	Baked and refried beans
Asparagus	Beans, all	Breaded, fried, deep-fried, or sautéed vegetables
Bamboo shoots	Corn	Olives, packed in oil
Beets and beet greens	Lentils	Potatoes, white
Beans (green and yellow wax)	Sweet potatoes	Sweet pickles
Bok choy	Peas (split, black-eyed)	
Broccoflower	Potatoes (purple, red)	
Broccoli	Yams	
Broccoli rabe		
Broccolini		
Brussels sprouts		
Cabbage (Chinese, green, red, savoy)		
Carrots		

VEGETABLES AND LEGUMES

Choose Prepare raw, lightly steamed, or grilled	Limit until you reach your weight-loss goal	Avoid
Cassava		
Cauliflower		
Celery		
Celeriac		
Chard		
Chayote		
Collards		
Cucumber		
Dandelion greens		
Eggplant		
Endive		
Fennel		
Jicama		
Kale		
Kohlrabi		
Lettuce, all varieties		
Mushrooms, all varieties		
Mustard greens		
Okra		
Onions		
Parsley		
Pea pods		
Peppers (red, green, yellow, purple)		
Radicchio		

VEGETABLES AND LEGUMES		
Choose *Prepare raw, lightly steamed, or grilled*	**Limit** *until you reach your weight-loss goal*	**Avoid**
Radishes, all varieties		
Rutabaga		
Sauerkraut		
Scallions		
Sorrel		
Soybeans (edamame, organic only)		
Spinach		
Sprouts		
Squash (Hubbard, spaghetti, summer/ yellow, zucchini)		
Tomatillo		
Tomato (though considered a vegetable, is actually a fruit, classified a berry), all varieties		
Taro		
Turnips		
Water chestnuts		
Watercress		

FRUITS	
Choose	**Avoid**
Apple	Banana
Apricot	Candied fruit
Blackberries	Canned fruit
Blueberries	Dried fruit

FRUITS	
Choose	**Avoid**
Cantaloupe	Grapes, all types
Cherries	Mango
Coconut	Persimmons
Grapefruit	Plantain
Honeydew	Raisins
Kiwi	Watermelon
Melon	
Nectarine	
Orange	
Papaya	
Peach	
Pear	
Pineapple	
Plum	
Raspberries	
Strawberries	
Tangelo	
Tangerine	

PROTEIN		
	Choose	**Avoid**
Vegan	**Animal** *Prepare baked, broiled, grilled, or steamed*	**Animal** *Completely avoid all breaded, fried, and deep-fried foods*
Beans	Beef: lean cuts are best, such as flank, ground beef (less than 10 percent fat), New York strip, sirloin, tenderloin, top round	Beef, all fatty cuts, more toxins are stored in fat than muscle)

PROTEIN		
Choose		**Avoid**
Lentils	Bison (buffalo)	Bacon
Organic tofu (in small amounts)	Calamari	Buffalo wings
Nuts	Chicken (skinless breast and thighs are best)	Canadian bacon
Split peas	Clams	Fish sticks
	Cornish game hen	Fried chicken
	Crab	Ground beef (greater than 10 percent fat)
	Eggs	Hot dogs (beef, chicken, pork, turkey)
	Elk	Jerky, beef and turkey
	Fresh wild-caught fish, all types	Liver
	Lamb	Liverwurst
	Mussels	Pork (especially bacon and honey-baked ham)
	Oysters	Processed poultry products
	Turkey (skinless is best)	Salami
	Turkey bacon (limit two slices)	Sausage
		Seafood (canned in oil)
		Turkey bacon
		Turkey sausage

DAIRY AND DAIRY ALTERNATIVES	
Choose *antibiotic-free, preferably organic*	**Avoid**
Alternative milk (almond, hemp, oak, rice)	Cottage cheese

DAIRY AND DAIRY ALTERNATIVES	
Choose *antibiotic-free, preferably* *organic*	**Avoid**
Cheese (best choices are almond, feta, goat, rice)	Cream, half-and-half
	Cream cheese, all types
	Frozen yogurt
	Ice cream, all types
	Milk
	Most cheese (except for Choose list)
	Sour cream
	Yogurt

BEVERAGES	
Choose	**Avoid**
Green tea	Alcohol (beer, wine, mixed drinks)
Herbal tea	Beverages with artificial flavors or sweeteners
Mineral water with lemon, lime, or unsweetened cranberry concentrate for flavor	Beverages with sugar, high-fructose corn syrup, or other sweeteners
Vegetable juices	Chocolate drinks, cocoa
White tea	Coffee
	Diet sodas
	Flavored water, sweetened
	Fruit juices
	Sodas
	Soy milk (a goitrogen)
	Sports drinks

GRAINS, BREADS, AND CEREALS	
Choose	Avoid
100 percent sprouted whole grain	Bagels, all types
Barley	Biscuits
Brown rice	Bread (except for Choose list)
Buckwheat groats	Bread crumbs
Muesli (no sugar or dried fruit added)	Bread sticks
Oat bran	Chips, all types
Oat bran bread	Corn bread
Oatmeal, steel cut	Crackers, all types
Rice bran	Croissants
Rye, whole	English muffins
Unsweetened bran cereals	Granola, all types, and other cereals (except for Choose list)
Wild rice (cereal grass)	Melba toast
	Muffins, all types
	Pancakes
	Pasta and noodles, including ramen style
	Pita bread
	Popcorn (until you reach your goal weight)
	Popcorn cakes
	Pretzels
	Rice (white, fried, Spanish)
	Rice cakes
	Rolls (dinner rolls; hamburger, hot dog buns)
	Soups (cream-based, noodle, pasta types)
	Taco shells

GRAINS, BREADS, AND CEREALS

Choose	Avoid
	Tortillas
	Waffles

FATS AND OILS

Choose	Avoid
Coconut oil (virgin, organic)	Canola oil
Olive oil (extra virgin, organic)	Corn oil
	Peanut oil
	Safflower oil
	Soybean oil
	Sunflower oil

NUTS, NUT BUTTERS, SEEDS, AND SEED BUTTERS

Item	Amount
Almond butter	1 tsp.
Almonds	Less than 24
Brazil nuts	Less than 6
Cashew butter	1 tsp.
Cashews	Less than 6
Hazelnut butter	1 tsp.
Hazelnuts	Less than 12
Macadamia nut butter	1 tsp.
Macadamia nuts	Less than 12
Pecan halves	Less than 24
Pine nuts	Less than 24
Pistachios	Less than 24
Pumpkin seeds	Less than 2 Tbsp.
Sesame seeds	Less than 2 Tbsp.
Sunflower seeds	Less than 2 Tbsp.
Tahini (sesame seed butter)	1 tsp.
Walnut halves	Less than 12

SUGAR, SUGAR SUBSTITUTES, AND SWEET TREATS

Choose	Avoid
Fresh fruit	Agave syrup*
Frozen coconut water	Artificial sweeteners, all
Seeds (sunflower, pumpkin)	Brown rice syrup*
	Brown sugar
	Brownies
	Cakes
	Candy
	Candy bars
	Cane juice
	Chocolate
	Cookies
	Corn syrup
	Dextrin
	Doughnuts
	Energy bars
	Frozen treats
	Frozen yogurt
	Gelatin
	High-fructose corn syrup
	Raw honey*
	Ice cream
	Maple syrup, pure*
	Molasses
	Mousse
	Pastries
	Pies
	Pudding

SUGAR, SUGAR SUBSTITUTES, AND SWEET TREATS	
Choose	Avoid
	Sorbet
	Sucanat
	Sucrose (white sugar)
	Sugar alcohols (i.e., sorbitol, manitol)
	Tofu frozen dessert
	Whipped topping
	Xylitol

*These are OK if used very sparingly. But avoid them whenever possible because they do contain sugar.

CONDIMENTS	
Choose	Avoid
Extra-virgin olive oil	Bacon bits
Garlic	Commercial salad dressings made with polyunsaturated oils
Herbs	Croutons
Horseradish	Fruit jams, jellies, marmalades, preserves
Hummus	Fruit sauces
Lemon juice	Ketchup
Lime juice	Lard
Mayonnaise	Margarine
Mustard	Peanut butter
Olives, packed in water	Pickles (except dill)
Onions	Sandwich spreads
Pickles, dill	Shortening, vegetable
Salsa	Sour cream
Sauerkraut	Sweet pickle relish
Shallots	

CONDIMENTS	
Choose	Avoid
Spaghetti sauce, sugar free	
Spices	
Tahini	
Virgin coconut oil	

Guidelines for Servings Per Day

- Protein—animal or vegan: 4-6 ounces per meal
- Eggs—no more than one per day
- Legumes—three 1-cup servings per week
- Grains—two to three 1-cup servings per week
- Nuts, seeds, nut butters—twenty-four small seeds; twelve medium size such as almonds; six large nuts such as macadamia; 1 teaspoon nut butter
- Fruit—one or two servings per day
- Vegetables—unlimited
- Sweetener—small amount of stevia

NOTES

1—WEIGHT LOSS ON A MISSION

1. As referenced in Antoaneta Sawyer, "Role of Probiotics and Prebiotics in the Modern Diet," Examiner.com, June 12, 2010, http://www .examiner.com/diets-in-milwaukee/role-of-probiotics-and-prebiotics-the-modern-diet (accessed March 9, 2011).

2. *First for Women*, "Dr. Oz's #1 Fat Cure," January 10, 2011, 32–35.

3. Patrice Carter, Laura J. Gray, Jacqui Troughton, Kamlesh Khunti, and Melanie J. Davies, "Fruit and Vegetable Intake and Incidence of Type 2 Diabetes Mellitus: Systematic Review and Meta-Analysis," *British Medical Journal* 341 (August 2010): http://www.bmj.com/content/341/ bmj.c4229.full (accessed March 8, 2011).

4. Adein Cassidy et al., "Plasma Adiponectin Concentrations Are Associated With Body Composition and Plant-Based Dietary Factors in Female Twins," *Journal of Nutrition* 139, no. 2 (February 2009): 353–358.

5. ScienceDaily.com, "Brain Chemical Boosts Body Heat, Aids in Calorie Burn, UT Southwestern Research Suggests," July 7, 2010, http://www .sciencedaily.com/releases/2010/07/100706123015.htm (accessed March 6, 2011).

6. ScienceDaily.com, "Peppers May Increase Energy Expenditure in People Trying to Lose Weight," April 28, 2010, http://www.sciencedaily .com/releases/2010/04/100427190934.htm (accessed December 28, 2010).

7. Judy Siegel, "Garlic Prevents Obesity," *Jerusalem Post*, October 30, 2001, 5.

8. Niki Fears, "Cranberries and Weight Loss," eHow.com, http://www .ehow.com/about_5417851_cranberries-weight-loss.html (accessed December 28, 2010).

9. *Woman's World*, "Slimming New Juice Cure," December 27, 2010, 18–19.

10. ScienceDaily.com, "Blueberries May Help Reduce Belly Fat, Diabetes Risk," April 20, 2009, http://www.sciencedaily.com/ releases/2009/04/090419170112.htm (accessed March 9, 2011).

11. Jennie Brand-Miller, "A Glycemic Index Expert Responds to the Tufts Research," DiabetesHealth.com, October 18, 2007, http://www

.diabeteshealth.com/read/2007/10/18/5496/a-glycemic-index-expert-responds-to-the-tufts-research (accessed February 5, 2010).

12. Richard Fogoros, "Low Glycemic Weight Loss Is Longer Lasting," About.com: Heart Disease, http://heartdisease.about.com/od/dietandobesity/a/logly.htm (accessed March 12, 2010).

2—TOP TEN ROADBLOCKS TO WEIGHT LOSS

1. A conversation Dr. Robert C. Atkins had with Brenda Watson, author of *Gut Solutions*, as related to Cherie Calbom by Brenda Watson, February 2004.

2. Craig Lambert, "Deep Into Sleep," *Harvard Magazine*, July–August 2005, http://harvardmagazine.com/2005/07/deep-into-sleep.html (accessed January 29, 2010).

3. National Sleep Foundation, *2005 Sleep in America Poll*, March 29, 2005, http://www.sleepfoundation.org/sites/default/files/2005_summary_of_findings.pdf (accessed January 29, 2010).

4. James E. Gangwisch, Dolores Malaspina, Bernadette Boden-Albala, and Steven B. Heymsfield, "Inadequate Sleep as a Risk Factor for Obesity: Analyses of the NHANES 1," *Sleep* 28, no. 10 (2005): 1289–1296, http://www.journalsleep.org/Articles/281017.pdf (accessed February 2, 2010).

5. Colette Bouchez, "The Dream Diet: Losing Weight While You Sleep," WebMD.com, http://www.webmd.com/sleep-disorders/guide/lose-weight-while-sleeping (accessed March 10, 2011).

6. John Easton, "Lack of Sleep Alters Hormones, Metabolism," *University of Chicago Chronicle*, December 2, 1999, http://chronicle.uchicago.edu/991202/sleep.shtml (accessed March 10, 2011).

7. Bouchez, "The Dream Diet: Losing Weight While You Sleep."

8. Ibid.

9. Easton, "Lack of Sleep Alters Hormones, Metabolism."

10. Cherie Calbom and John Calbom, *Sleep Away the Pounds* (New York: Warner Wellness, 2007).

11. Ulrich Harttig and George S. Bailey, "Chemoprotection by Natural Chlorophylls *in vivo*: Inhibition of Dibenzo[*a,l*]pyrene–DNA Adducts in Rainbow Trout Liver," *Carcinogenesis* 19, no. 7 (1998): 1323–1326.

12. Mercola.com, "The Truth About Candida Overgrowth," December 4, 2009, http://www.drmercola.info/2009/12/the-truth-about-candida

-overgrowth/ (accessed March 9, 2011).

13. R. E. Ley, P. J. Turnbaugh, S. Klein, and J. I. Gordon, "Microbial Ecology: Human Gut Microbes Associated With Obesity," *Nature* 444, no. 7122 (December 21, 2006): 1022–1023.

14. Y. Kadooka et al., "Regulation of Abdominal Adiposity by Probiotics (Lactobacillus gasseri SBT2055) in Adults With Obese Tendencies in a Randomized Controlled Trial," *European Journal of Clinical Nutrition* 64, no. 6 (June 2010): 636–643.

15. Katherine Zeratsky, "Probiotics: Important for a Healthy Diet?", MayoClinic.com, April 17, 2010, http://www.mayoclinic.com/health/probiotics/AN00389 (accessed March 9, 2011).

16. *First for Women*, "Break the Yeast–Belly Fat Cycle," 31.

17. D. O. Ogbolu, A. A. Oni, O. A. Daini, and A. P. Oloko, "*In Vitro* Antimicrobial Properties of Coconut Oil on Candida Species in Ibadan, Nigeria," *Journal of Medical Food* 10, no. 2 (June 2007): 384–387.

18. Joseph Mercola, "This Cooking Oil Is a Powerful Virus-Destroyer and Antibiotic…," Mercola.com, October 22, 2010, http://articles.mercola.com/sites/articles/archive/2010/10/22/coconut-oil-and-saturated-fats-can-make-you-healthy.aspx (accessed March 9, 2011).

19. Ibid.

3—Why a Liquid Diet Jump-Starts Weight Loss

1. Megan Rauscher, "Vegetable Juice May Help With Weight Loss," Reuters.com, April 22, 2009, http://www.reuters.com/article/idUSTRE53L60S20090422 (accessed February 5, 2010).

2. MedicalNewsToday.com, "Vegetable Use Aided in Dietary Support for Weight Loss and Lower Blood Pressure," October 21, 2009, http://www.medicalnewstoday.com/articles/168174.php (accessed February 5, 2010).

3. Ibid.

4. Ibid.

5. WebMD.com, "What Is Metabolic Syndrome?" January 25, 2009, http://www.webmd.com/heart/metabolic-syndrome/metabolic-syndrome-what-is-it (accessed January 27, 2010).

6. PRNewswire.com, "How Much Do Fruits and Vegetables Really Cost?", February 3, 2011, http://www.prnewswire.com/news-releases/how-much-do-fruits-and-vegetables-really-cost-115223374.html (accessed March 9, 2011).

4—THE WEEKEND WEIGHT-LOSS DIET

1. National Weight Control Registry, "NWCR Facts," http://www.nwcr .ws/Research/default.htm (accessed March 9, 2011).

2. "Dr. Oz's Top 5 Mistakes Dieters Make," posted by Norine Dworkin-McDaniel, ThatsFit.com, December 26, 2010, http://www.thatsfit.com /2010/12/26/dr-ozs-top-5-mistakes-dieters-make/ (accessed March 9, 2011).

3. Mark A. Pereira, Janis Swain, Allison B. Goldfine, Nader Rifai, and David S. Ludwig, "Effects of a Low-Glycemic Load Diet on Resting Energy Expenditure and Heart Disease Risk Factors During Weight Loss," *Journal of the American Medical Association* 292, no. 20 (November 24, 2004): 2482–2490.

5—IN THE PRODUCE AISLE (SHOPPING GUIDE)

1. Virginia Worthington, "Nutritional Quality of Organic Versus Conventional Fruits, Vegetables, and Grains," *Journal of Alternative and Complementary Medicine* 7, no. 2 (2001): 161–173.

2. Joseph Mercola with Rachel Droege, "How Many Pesticides Are in Your Food? Find Out Now!", March 10, 2004, http://articles.mercola .com/sites/articles/archive/2004/03/10/pesticides-food.aspx (accessed March 9, 2011).

3. Maryland Pesticide Network, "Pesticide News," http://www.mdpestnet .org/resource/news/2010.htm (accessed February 7, 2010).

4. Melissa J. Perry and Frederick R. Bloom, "Perceptions of Pesticide-Associated Cancer Risks Among Farmers: A Qualitative Assessment," *Human Organization* 57 (1998): 342–349.

5. Maria Rodale "Organic Can Feed the World," *PCC Sound Consumer*, September 2010.

6. Ibid.

7. Jon Ungoed-Thomas, "Official: Organic Really Is Better," *Sunday Times*, October 28, 2007, http://www.timesonline.co.uk/tol/news/uk/ health/article2753446.ece (accessed January 28, 2010).

8. Worthington, "Nutritional Quality of Organic Versus Conventional Fruits, Vegetables, and Grains"; US Department of Agriculture, *Pesticide Data Program: Annual Summary Calendar Year 2005* (Washington: Agricultural Marketing Service, 2006), http://www.ams .usda.gov/AMSv1.0/getfile?dDocName=STELPRDC5049946 (accessed February 3, 2011).

9. Jeffrey Norris, "Chemicals in Environment Deserve Study for Possible Role in Fat Gain, Says Byers Award Recipient," UCSF News, December 15, 2010, http://www.ucsf.edu/news/2010/12/6017/obesity-pesticides -pollutants-toxins-and-drugs-linked-studies-c-elegans (accessed March 10, 2011).

10. Ronnie Cummins, "The Road Ahead: Steps Toward a Global Uprising," Organic Consumers Association, December 9, 2010, http://www .organicconsumers.org/articles/article_22174.cfm (accessed March 11, 2011). Also, Environmental Working Group, "EWG's Shopper's Guide to Pesticides in Produce," http://www.ewg.org/foodnews/summary/ (accessed October 20, 2011).

11. US Food and Drug Administration, "Regulation of Foods Derived From Plants," statement of Lester M. Crawford before the Subcommittee on Conservation, Rural Development, and Research House Committee on Agriculture, June 17, 2003, http://www.fda.gov/ NewsEvents/Testimony/ucm161037.htm (accessed March 11, 2011).

12. Mavis Butcher, "Genetically Modified Food—GM Foods List and Information," Disabled-World.com, September 22, 2009 http://www .disabled-world.com/fitness/gm-foods.php (accessed March 11, 2011).

13. Ibid.

14. What's on My Food?, "51 Pesticide Residues Found by the USDA Pesticide Data Program," http://www.whatsonmyfood.org/food .jsp?food=LT (accessed October 20, 2011).

15. Environmental Working Group, "EWG's Shopper's Guide to Pesticides in Produce," http://www.ewg.org/foodnews/summary/ (accessed October 20, 2011).

16. J. D. Decuypere, "Radiation, Irradiation, and Our Food Supply," *The Decuypere Report*, http://www.healthalternatives2000.com/food -supply-report.html (accessed March 11, 2011).

17. Ibid.

18. Ibid.

19. US Food and Drug Administration, "Regulation of Foods Derived From Plants," statement of Lester M. Crawford before the Subcommittee on Conservation, Rural Development, and Research House Committee on Agriculture, June 17, 2003, http://www.fda.gov/ NewsEvents/Testimony/ucm161037.htm (accessed March 11, 2011).

20. Mavis Butcher, "Genetically Modified Food—GM Foods List and

Information," Disabled-World.com, September 22, 2009 http://www
.disabled-world.com/fitness/gm-foods.php (accessed March 11, 2011).

21. Ibid.

22. Ronnie Cummins, "The Road Ahead: Steps Toward a Global Uprising,"
Organic Consumers Association, December 9, 2010, http://www
.organicconsumers.org/articles/article_22174.cfm (accessed March 11,
2011).

6—Beyond the Weekend: How to Keep Losing Weight and Feeling Great

1. EatWild.com, "Summary of Important Health Benefits of Grassfed
Meats, Eggs, and Dairy," http://www.eatwild.com/healthbenefits.htm
(accessed February 3, 2010).

2. C. Ip, J. A. Scimeca, and H. J. Thompson, "Conjugated Linoleic Acid: A
Powerful Anticarcinogen From Animal Fat Sources," *Cancer* 74, suppl.
3 (August 1, 1994): 1050–1054; K. L. Houseknecht, J. P. Vanden Heuvel,
S. Y. Moya-Camarena, et al., "Dietary Conjugated Linoleic Acid
Normalizes Impaired Glucose Tolerance in the Zucker Diabetic Fatty
Fa/Fa Rat," *Biochemical and Biophysical Research Communications*
244, no. 3 (March 27, 1998): 678–682, abstract viewed at http://www
.ncbi.nlm.nih.gov/pubmed/9535724 (accessed February 3, 2010).

3. G. C. Smith, "Dietary Supplementation of Vitamin E to Cattle
to Improve Shelf Life and Case Life of Beef for Domestic and
International Markets," Colorado State University, referenced in
EatWild.com, "Summary of Important Health Benefits of Grassfed
Meats, Eggs, and Dairy," http://www.eatwild.com/healthbenefits.htm
(accessed March 11, 2011).

4. W. G. Kruggel, R. A. Field, G. J. Miller, K. M. Horton, and J. R.
Busboom, "Influence of Sex and Diet on Lutein in Lamb Fat," *Journal
of Animal Science* 54 (1982): 970–975.

5. World-wire.com, "American Public Health Association Supports
Ban on Hormonal Milk and Meat," news release, November 13, 2009,
http://www.world-wire.com/news/0911130001.html (accessed March
11, 2011).

6. ConsumerReports.org. "Chicken: Arsenic and Antibiotics," July 2007,
http://www.consumerreports.org/cro/food/food-safety/animal-feed
-and-food/animal-feed-and-the-food-supply-105/chicken-arsenic-and
-antibiotics/index.htm (accessed March 11, 2011).

7. Tabitha Alterman, "Eggciting News!" MotherEarthNews.com, October 15, 2008, http://www.motherearthnews.com/Relish/Pastured-Eggs -Vitamin-D-Content.aspx (accessed March 11, 2011).

8. Ibid.

9. L. Scalfi, A. Coltorti, and F. Contaldo, "Postprandial Thermogenesis in Lean and Obese Subjects After Meals Supplemented With Medium-Chain and Long-Chain Triglycerides," *American Journal of Clinical Nutrition* 53, no. 5 (May 1, 1991): 1130–1133.

10. Ogbolu, Oni, Daini, and Oloko, "*In Vitro* Antimicrobial Properties of Coconut Oil on Candida Species in Ibadan, Nigeria."

11. "Vegetable Oils/Fatty Acid Composition, Hexane Residues, Declaration, Pesticides (Organic Culinary Oils Only)," a joint campaign Basel city (specialist laboratory) and Basel county, http://www.kantonslabor-bs. ch/files/berichte/Report0424.pdf (accessed March 11, 2011).

12. S. Couvreur, C. Hurtaud, C. Lopez, L. Delaby, and J. L. Peyraud, "The Linear Relationship Between the Proportion of Fresh Grass in the Cow Diet, Milk Fatty Acid Composition, and Butter Properties," *Journal of Dairy Science* 89, no. 6 (June 2006): 1956–1969, as referenced in EatWild.com, "Summary of Important Health Benefits of Grassfed Meats, Eggs, and Dairy."

13. Ibid.

14. S. O'Keefe, S. Gaskins-Wright, V. Wiley, and I-C. Chen, "Levels of Trans Geometrical Isomers of Essential Fatty Acids in Some Unhydrogenated U.S. Vegetable Oils," *Journal of Food Lipids* 1, no. 3 (September 1994): 165–176, referenced in WestonAPrice.org, "The Oiling of America," January 1, 2000, http://www.westonaprice.org/ know-your-fats/525-the-oiling-of-america.html (accessed March 11, 2011).

15. *New York Times*, "Fat in Margarine Is Tied to Heart Problems," May 16, 1994, http://www.nytimes.com/1994/05/16/us/fat-in-margarine-is -tied-to-heart-problems.html (accessed March 11, 2011).

16. Alice Park, "Can Sugar Substitutes Make You Fat?" *Time*, February 10, 2008, http://www.time.com/time/health/article/0,8599,1711763,00.html (accessed March 11, 2011).

17. Woodrow C. Monte, "Aspartame: Methanol and Public Health," *Journal of Applied Nutrition* 36, no. 1 (1984): 44, referenced in documentary *Sweet Misery* (Tucson, AZ: Sound and Fury Productions,

2004), http://www.soundandfury.tv/pages/sweet%20misery.html (accessed March 11, 2011).

18. Ibid., also, Dani Veracity, "The Link Between Aspartame and Brain Tumors: What the FDA Never Told You About Artificial Sweeteners," NaturalNews.com, September 22, 2005, http://www.naturalnews .com/011804.html (accessed March 11, 2011).

19. Citizens for Health, "Chairman of Citizens for Health Declares FDA Should Review Approval of Splenda," press release, September 22, 2008, http://www.globenewswire.com/newsroom/news.html?d=150785 (accessed March 11, 2011), referenced in Joanne Waldron, "Duke University Study Links Splenda to Weight Gain, Health Problems," NaturalNews.com, October 20, 2008, http://www.naturalnews .com/024543.html (accessed March 11, 2011).

20. Byron Richards, "High Fructose Corn Syrup Makes Your Brain Crave Food," 51commerce.net, April 1, 2009, http://www.51commerce.net/ weight/articles/high_fructose_corn_syrup_makes_your_brain_crave_ food/index.htm (accessed March 11, 2011).

21. Yoshio Nagai et al., "The Role of Peroxisome Proliferator-Activated Receptor γ Coactivator-1 β in the Pathogenesis of Fructose-Induced Insulin Resistance," Cell Metabolism 9, no. 3 (March 4, 2009): 252–264.

22. International Journal of Obesity and Related Metabolic Disorders (September 16, 2003), referenced in "Calcium and Weight Loss," In Focus Newsletter, May 2005, http://www.nutricology.com/In-Focus -Newsletter-May-2005-sp-45.html (accessed February 4, 2010).

23. Y. C. Lin, R. M. Lyle, L. D. McCabe, G. P. McCabe, C. M. Weaver, and D. Teegarden, "Daily Calcium Is Related to Changes in Body Composition During a Two-Year Exercise Intervention in Young Women," Journal of the American College of Nutrition 19, no 6 (November–December 2000): 754–760, abstract viewed at http://www .ncbi.nlm.nih.gov/pubmed/11194528 (accessed February 4, 2010).

24. K. M. Davies, R. P. Heaney, R. R. Recker, et al., "Calcium Intake and Body Weight," Journal of Clinical Endocrinology and Metabolism 85, no. 12 (December 2000): 4635–4638, abstract viewed at http://www .ncbi.nlm.nih.gov/pubmed/11134120 (accessed February 4, 2010).

25. Endocrine Today, "High Levels of Vitamin D, Low-Calorie Diet May Increase Weight Loss," December 31, 2009, http://www.endocrinetoday .com/view.aspx?rid=59663 (accessed February 4, 2010).

26. F. Ceci, C. Cangiano, M. Cairella, et al., "The Effects of Oral 5-Hydroxytryptophan Administration on Feeding Behavior in Obese Adult Female Subjects," *Journal of Neural Transmission* 76, no. 2 (1989): 109–117.

27. C. Cangiano, F. Ceci, M. Cairella, et al., "Effects of 5-Hydroxytryptophan on Eating Behavior and Adherence to Dietary Prescriptions in Obese Adult Subjects," *Advances in Experimental Medicine and Biology* 294 (1991): 591–593.

28. Steven A. Abrams, Ian J. Griffin, Keli M. Hawthorne, and Kenneth J. Ellis, "Effect of Prebiotic Supplementation and Calcium Intake on Body Mass Index," *Journal of Pediatrics* 151, no. 3 (September 2007): 293–298, abstract viewed at http://www.jpeds.com/article/S0022-3476(07)00280-6/abstract (accessed February 4, 2010).

29. USAToday.com, "Study: 10 Minutes of Exercise Yields Hour-Long Effects," June 1, 2010, http://www.usatoday.com/news/health/weightloss/2010-06-01-exercise-metabolism_N.htm (accessed March 9, 2011).

30. Ibid.

31. Calbom and Calbom, *Sleep Away the Pounds.*

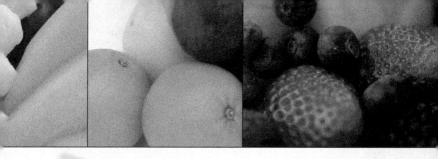

More books from the Juice Lady...

Eat your way to *health*, *detoxification*, and *weight loss*

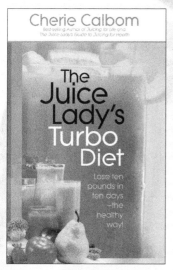

978-1-61638-149-3 / $17.99

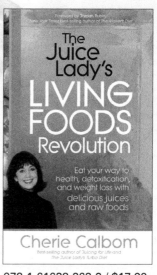

978-1-61638-363-3 / $17.99

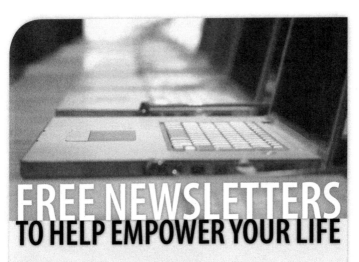